KNOWING YOUR PARENTS

- ☐ **Diary Entry**
- ☐ **View Points**
- ☐ **Counsellor's Advice**

Author
Seema Gupta

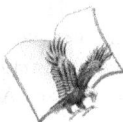

V&S PUBLISHERS

Published by:

V&S PUBLISHERS

F-2/16, Ansari Road, Daryaganj, New Delhi-110002
☎ 011-23240026, 011-23240027 • *Fax:* 011-23240028
Email: info@vspublishers.com • *Website:* www.vspublishers.com

Regional Office : Hyderabad
5-1-707/1, Brij Bhawan (Beside Central Bank of India Lane)
Bank Street, Koti, Hyderabad - 500 095
☎ 040-24737290
E-mail: vspublishershyd@gmail.com

Branch Office : Mumbai
Jaywant Industrial Estate, 2nd Floor–222, Tardeo Road
Opposite Sobo Central Mall, Mumbai – 400 034
☎ 022-23510736
E-mail vspublishersmum@gmail.com

Follow us on: 🇹 f in

All books available at www.vspublishers.com

Printed at : Repro Knowledgecast Limited, Thane

Publisher's Note

At V&S Publishers, it has been our constant endeavour to bring forth books which are rich in content, affordably priced and ever so interesting. This book, however, is a special effort by us to contribute to the society we live in. Through this unique piece of work, thoughtfully and beautifully carved out by our respected author, Seema Gupta, we sincerely hope to resolve the conflict between the teenagers and their parents, particularly in our Indian society, as we feel that unlike the Western countries, our society, in terms of its new interests and diverse exposure is still in its nascent stages and teenagers need to make a constant and continuous effort to bridge this generation gap which has become more prominent over the last decade with the Western culture seeping in.

Parenting or rearing children, especially during their teens, is indeed a tough and challenging job! These are the years when there is a complete mental and physical transformation in a child's personality and behaviour. As children step out from their long period of completely sheltered childhood, they start feeling independent with their own set of ideas, values, whims and fancies, and likes and dislikes. They begin to develop their individual thinking and perceptions.

With children needing to take big decisions regarding their future and career, teenage thus, furthermore becomes a crucial period. The problem, however, arises due to constant conflict in interests and opinions of teenagers and parents with both being right and wrong at the same time in their own perspectives.

Keeping in mind our Indian society and in view of this ever rising problem of 'Knowing Your Parent', the author in this book has uniquely presented the views and grievances of the parents in the form of interesting and simple Diary Entry. These entries have been accompanied with a Counsellor's advice which gives the required advice to the teenager and his or her parent depending upon the issue concerned. This further gives a third person perspective to the addressed problem and proposes a feasible solution to the whole conflict.

We all are aware that there develops a generation gap between parents and children as they grow up and step into their teens. This gap has to be bridged by some deep thinking and understanding, by they child. Teenagers should respect the feelings and aspirations of their parents. The author suggests that they should sit together as often as they can, just as friends, and discuss their viewpoints, problems, etc., and also debate on them, if required in a healthy atmosphere and then reach to an amicable consensus or solution.

We hope the book will serve the purpose effectively and compel our readers to go through it again and again, irrespective of their age, colour, sex or cultural background and hopefully will act as a handbook for teenagers' reference during conflicting scenarios.

Preface

The adolescents and young adults form that salient section of our vast and diverse society which is perplexed about their own position, for their age group is neither too big to be called a fully matured individual, nor too small to be called as children.

Generally, the mindset of the adolescents is that parents are not their well-wishers. They are old-fashioned, rigid and dominating. This may be true sometimes and in certain cases, but not always. The youngsters feel that parents are good till they 'give in' and the moment they don't, they are *numero uno* enemy, which, they are certainly not.

However, the levels of stress that the adolescents face these days, at times does go beyond the comprehension of an adult mind. With modern electronic gadgets chipping in almost every other day, the lifestyle of the youngsters have completely transformed from what it was when their parents were teenagers. For example, an account on Facebook, today is considered to be a must to fit in their circle of friends. Calling each other is passe, the youngsters either chat on these sites or sms through their mobiles.

This may be difficult for the parents to comprehend as there is a big generation gap which needs to be bridged by sheer patience, faith and understanding on the part of both the parties.

In this book are given some *Diary Entry* from the diary of the parents. Who are marred with the problem, and try to resolve it in their own inimitable ways. Each diary entry is assessed and followed by a *Counsellor's Advice* which provides an amicable solution to the concerned problem in an unbiased manner.

Contents

1

Late Night Parties

Late night parties for teenagers are not acceptable in most Indian households, especially if the teenager is a girl. Does this mean the parents are too orthodox or is there any reasonable explanation to this rule that teenagers find so appalling?

Let's visit Malhotra household and see what Anushka and her parents say in this matter.

The middle class Malhotra household has following members :

Anushka – 16-years old teenager (student of class X)

Rajesh – Anushka's father (employed in a marketing job)

Suruchi – Anushka's mother (housewife)

Abhinav – Anushka's brother (12-year old, student of class VII)

THE CONFLICT!!!

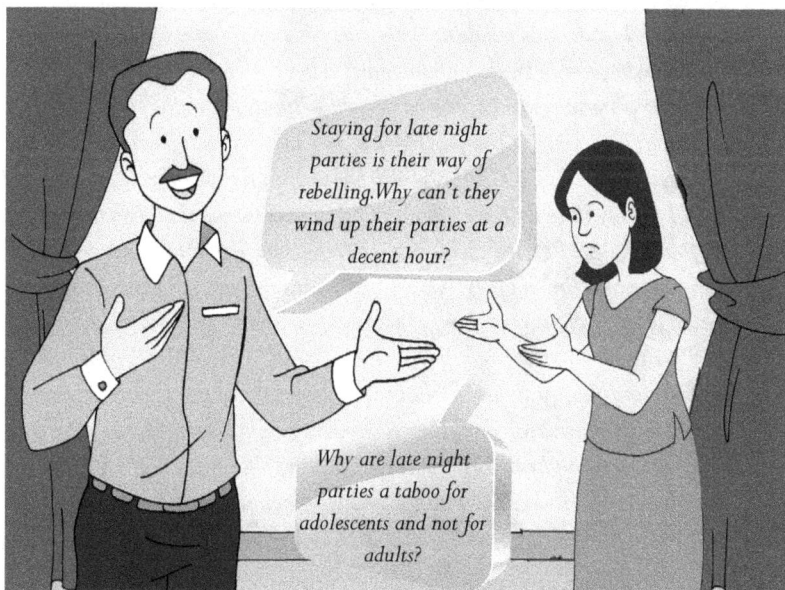

Staying for late night parties is their way of rebelling. Why can't they wind up their parties at a decent hour?

Why are late night parties a taboo for adolescents and not for adults?

Diary of Anushka's Mother

Monday, September 26, after dinner

Tonight over dinner, Anu told me about Jenny's party on Friday. She was quite forthright about wanting to go to this party which is likely to go beyond her deadline of 8 pm. When I tried to make her see reason that such parties are not acceptable she seemed to get into a bad mood and started sulking. She complained about the parties we organise and how boring she finds them. She insisted that she's a grown up girl now, soon she will be going to college. So how could we possibly force her to coop up in her own little world and not allow her to enjoy like others do. How do I make her understand that this enjoyment does not come without its share of risks?

She feels that she is an outcast in her group because we do not allow her to go for late night parties. But what she does not realise is that we do it for her own safety. The world is not so safe and people are not so trustworthy. Coming back from a party so late at night invites many bad elements leading to dire consequences. So why get into all this when it can be avoided at the base level.

I know she studies in co-educational school where boys and girls study together. But in a party, there are not only your school friends but other people too. Just the other day, my kitty party friend Ramola told me about her niece who had been drugged at such a party. I don't categorise and say that Anu's group would also be like this. But as the night progresses, the unfriendly elements are on the rise and our instincts become more wild leaving the civilised norms which we tend to follow otherwise. Why should I put my little daughter through all this while she is still so naïve?

Anu finds the parties we throw very boring and uncool because they begin early and finish early. Also I insist that from her friends' group only girls or some boys whom we know from their childhood should come. Instead, to make our party lively, I call a select group of our relatives and family friends whom we know and trust for long. But she loathes the idea of mingling her friends and our group. I never gave it much thought before because I always felt that children learn from their parents and I wanted my kids to socialise and learn to be

comfortable with people of all age groups and not just with their own group. But now that she tells me that she does not like it, I will try to amend it and may be let her have only her teenagers' party once in a while without inviting my own friends or relatives to it. We can always call them over some other day. But rules still remain the same.
No late nights.

Anu does not understand the extent of our love for her. Rajesh worries about the safety of Anu as well as of her friends and that is why he insists on personally dropping each and every girl of Anu's group who come to our place. This is to reciprocate the faith their parents posed in us when they sent their girls to our party and it is our duty that we drop them home safely on time.

Anu thinks deadline of 8 pm is way too early. But she does not understand the logic behind it. There are times when there is no one available to drop her home. Even Rajesh is on tour for better part of the month so he cannot go to fetch her. If she leaves the party at such earthly hour, then she can get public transport and even the roads are bustling with traffic, the chances of any mishap are minimal at this time as compared to 11 or 12 at night which is definitely not a safe hour for a girl travelling alone.

Another grievance of Anu's made me smile but I held it back. She thinks we are orthodox in our views and discriminate between girls and boys when it comes to giving liberties. She wanted to know if we would restrict Abhinav's party hours to 8 pm like hers. Oh yes, definitely. Safety is of paramount importance for everyone, be it a girl or a boy. Once he grows up and learns ways of life, then like Anu, he will also be free to lead his life.

As far as Anu is concerned, once she has become more mature and wise, we will set her free. But till then, she is our responsibility and we will try our best to protect her in every possible way.

I love my little girl and enjoy seeing her blossom like a rose. We may be acting like thorns around her but not to hurt her, just to protect her.

Suruchi

Counsellor Speaks

The problem between Anushka and her parents regarding late night parties stems from the root that many other girls are allowed to go to such parties, while Anushka's parents forbid her.

For Anushka

☐ It would help to allow Anushka to identify more such girls in her group who follow this norm of No Late Night Parties and not just compare herself with those who do not.

☐ Anushka may ask her friends who have been dropped by her father after her party, why they appreciate his gesture.

☐ Also she must have faith in her parents. They are her well-wishers, not her enemies. All that they have in their hearts is the thought of her safety and well-being. For that they have made many sacrifices and would always be willing to do so. So she should act mature now and understand the hidden thought behind all this curfew.

2

FB Fiasco

FB, Twitter, Google+, etc. are some of the popular social networking sites which are the craze among the youth today. But they are not as much in the good books of the parents.

Are the parents being the old duck or are their younglings overdoing this SNS bit?

Arjun lives in Chandigarh. He is like a normal youth of today whose life revolves around various networking sites. He has his own group of friends in school and an even bigger group of friends on Facebook. He loves interacting with them and spends a better part of his day on Internet. Let's meet Arjun and his family and see what they feel in this matter.

Members in Arjun's family

Arjun - 19 years old (student of class XII)
Surinder Ahuja – Arjun's father (self-employed, runs a grocery shop)
Radha – Arjun's mother (housewife)
Neha – Arjun's sister (16 years old, student of class X)

THE CONFLICT!!!

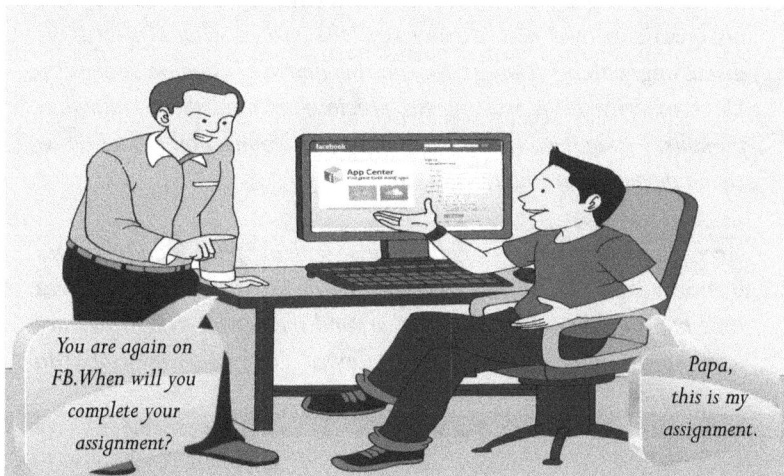

You are again on FB. When will you complete your assignment?

Papa, this is my assignment.

Diary of Arjun's Father

Monday, February 2, evening

Today, over lunch, I had a row with Arjun. When I went in to call him for dinner, I saw him sitting before the computer. And confirming my suspicions , the Facebook was on. I flew off my handle and scolded him left and right.

His exams are just round the corner and he is whiling away his time over these social networking sites. Isn't this outrageous? He has already flunked one year in this class. For how many years, do I have to continue paying his school fees and face the embarrassment of having a failure at home?

He claims that he flunked last year because he had chicken pox. I know that but if he had prepared well throughout the year, he would have managed to get passing marks in the physics paper. I went through hell of a trouble, got special permission from the school and board authorities so that he could write his paper in isolation. But he did not write it well because he had not prepared well.

Arjun says that chatting with his friends help him complete his projects and other assignments. I know it is all a cover up. Pray tell me, with his practicals over and exams round the corner, what project is he discussing with his friends? Most of his time is wasted on silly talks. Unnecessarily, he is wasting his precious time on these ridiculous pursuits. I even tried to remove the Internet connection but he threw such tantrums that I had to give in.

According to him when we can socialise with our friends and relatives then why is he not allowed to do so? We do socialise during our free time but not when the exams are around the corner. His exams are less than a month away. I have stopped going anywhere and do not entertain my guests at home so that Neha and Arjun do not get disturbed. Although Neha does not have board exams, thanks to the CCE pattern but at least Arjun should understand his responsibility.

His one big grouse is that I should also have my account on one of these social networking sites. He feels that if I have then I will understand them better. I do not see any logic into it. I know he only wants this because most of his friends' parents are on Facebook. It has become a kind of status symbol for him. But I see no reason how this will help him in studies. And in any case, where do I have the time to sit and chat on computer? I have my business to run from morning to night.

Arjun wants to be updated and in sync with times, and I have no objection to it. Thanks to God my shop is running well and I am able to provide a comfortable life to my family. That is why I bought him this laptop and got him an internet connection. But if he is going to misuse these facilities, then I would not hesitate in cutting down on the luxuries he is enjoying. It is as simple as this – you show me the result for the facilities I provide you.

Surinder

Counsellor Speaks

The problem between Arjun and his father is not just the difference of opinion, but it is also not understanding each other's viewpoint.

For Arjun

❐ Arjun has not been consistent in his studies, this is proved by the fact that he could not even get passing marks in his XII board exams, the previous year. His father ran from pillar to post, procured permission, so that he could write the papers when he was unwell, yet he could not pass. Naturally, his father is disappointed.

❐ Arjun is too much under peer pressure and that is why he is constantly comparing his father with the parents of his friends. Comparisons are never liked by anyone whether it is the young lot or the old. If he sincerely wants his father to understand the usefulness of social networking sites, he may ask his father to join him once in a while and see for himself how and what he does on Facebook.

❐ As for the moment, his father is right that Arjun should concentrate more on his studies instead of spending time on such pursuits.

3

Hole in My Pocket

While children like their pockets to be full all the time, parents worry that extra money may spoil the children.

Pocket money or no pocket money! This is one question which bothers both parents and kids alike, though for different reasons.

Meet Rajat and his father who have opposing views on the matter. Rajat lives in Delhi. He and his friends frequent nearby malls and have fun. This requires money and most of the time, Rajat somehow manages. But there are times when he gets stuck and feels embarrassed.

Members in Rajat's family :

Rajat — 16-year-old boy (student of class XI)
Tilak Singh- Rajat's father (bank employee)
Subhadra — Rajat's mother (school teacher)
Abhinav — Rajat's brother (9-year old)

THE CONFLICT!!!

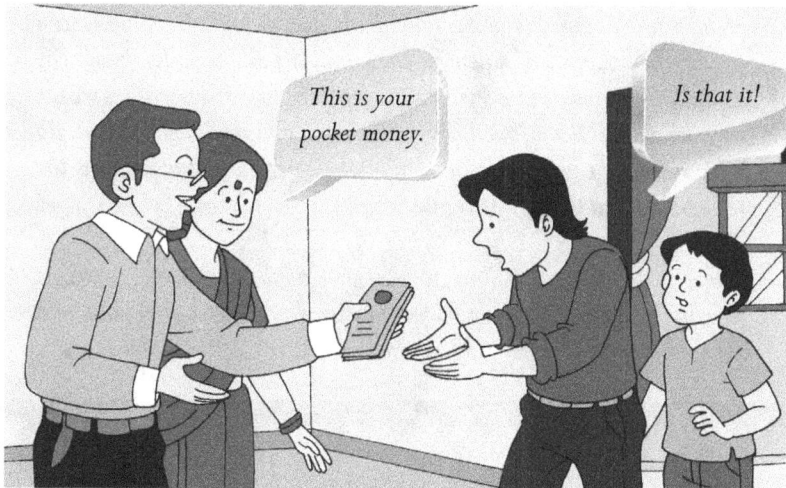

Diary of Rajat's Father

Rajat's exams finished yesterday. Today we were supposed to get the garage clean. When Rajat did not get up even till 10 am, I asked Subhadra. She told me that Rajat was very upset with me. It seems he was short of money yesterday and his friends had to pool in to pay for his movie ticket. I do not see why he feels so upset. If his pocket money cannot cover his expenses, then he should reduce his spending. We are a middle-class family. We have grown up valuing money and we want our children to do the same too.

I remember I used to get ten rupees per week for pocket money. I give Rajat one thousand bucks. Even that is not enough for him. I know inflation has gone up but it is upto us to spread our wings. I am sure he will spend even ten thousand rupees per month if I give him that amount. I want him to learn to save the money.

I can never forget what he did on his mother's birthday. He stole money from her wallet to give her present. When I rebuked him later, he had the cheek to tell me that it was I who instigated him to steal by not giving him enough pocket money. He refused to listen to reason. Seeing his stubborn attitude, I got angry and scolded him left and right. What I wanted to make him understand was that he should learn to plan his resources. When he knew that his mother's birthday was round the corner and he wanted to gift her expensive coffee maker then he should have saved his pocket money in advance. This would have been the true gift for his mother. It is not the gift alone, it is the thought behind that gift that matters.

Some of his friends belong to neo-rich families and their parents give them huge amounts of pocket money which they spend without a thought to it. But we are service class people. We cannot afford to give so much money to our children and spoil them.

These days Rajat has started a new drama. Whenever he wants a raise in his pocket money and I refuse to tow the line, then he threatens me that he would start working part time. Last November, he insisted on working at a stall in India International Trade Fair. I blankly refused. How could I allow him to lose fifteen days' school when exams were just round the corner? And what was the need? Really !

I wish someone could put some sense in his head and he should realise the importance of studies and value of money in life.

Tilak

Counsellor Speaks

Rajat and his father agree that Rajat should get pocket money, but they have totally different views when it comes to the amount of pocket money he should get.

For Rajat

❑ Rajat's father wants to inculcate good values in him. He feels that Rajat will not learn to value money if he gave him excess money. Rajat should not feel bad and respect his feelings.

❑ If Rajat had asked his father for money to buy a gift for his mother's birthday, he would not have refused. He should not have taken out money from his mother's wallet without asking her. This irked his father and placed the stigma of thief on him.

❑ Rajat should focus on his own life and not compare with some of his friends who are rich. He should come out of peer pressure and learn to think with his own mind

At Your Desk...

Studies are important in life. But is it necessary to spend most of the time to study or should there be a balance in studies and other activities? To answer this question, let us meet Sujata's family.

Sujata lives in Dehradun. Her mother is a single parent so she feels all the more responsible for her children. This makes her act unreasonably strict and sometimes even depresses her. This depression spreads to all the family members and the environment in the house becomes very suffocating.

There are three members in Sujata's family:

Sujata – 15-year-old girl (student of class IX)
Radhika Biyani – Sujata's mother(a government employee)
Gopal – Sujata's brother (18-year old student of class XII)

THE CONFLICT!!!

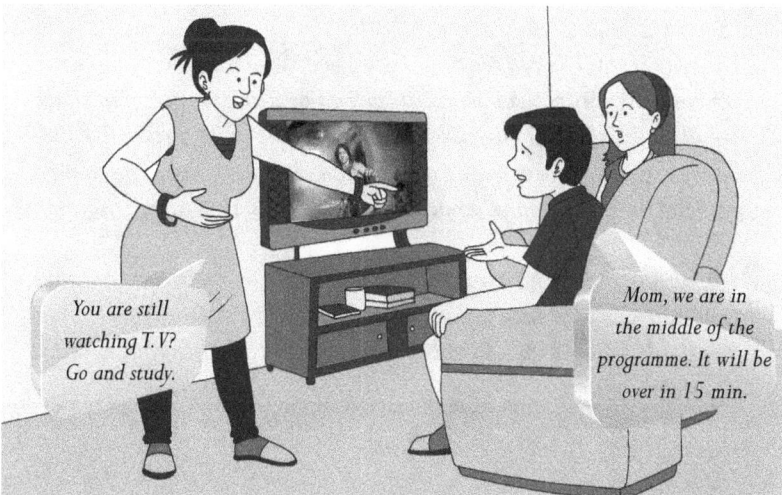

You are still watching T.V? Go and study.

Mom, we are in the middle of the programme. It will be over in 15 min.

Diary of Sujata's Mother

Tuesday, January 26, nightfall

I am so disappointed by both my children. As it is being a single parent is so difficult and then both Sujata and Gopal are not serious about their studies at all.

Since my husband Jai died four years ago, I have been fulfiling the responsibilities of both mother and father. I have given up all pleasures of life. I hardly go out and devote all my time to my children after office.

It hurts me when I see that they do not take their studies seriously. They should understand that life is not going to offer them goodies in a silver platter. They have to carve their own niche. No cajoling or scolding can make them see reason.

So long as I am around, they sit on their table with books in front of them, but the moment I turn around, they are either in front of TV or out with their friends. I even got the cable disconnected, so they would devote more time on studies. None of my children have mobile phones to distract them. Still their interest in studies is nil. They can hardly sit on their desk and concentrate on their books.

One day I found Sujata reading a story book which she kept within her course book. From the outside, it seemed as if she was deep in study, but actually, she was engrossed in a novel. The day I caught her red-handed all hell broke. Now I always look at her studies suspiciously. My God, how can young innocent children be so deceiving!

Gopal and Sujata have expressed their views many times that they would like to take the responsibility of their lives. How can I allow them to do so when they do not even understand the difference between right and wrong?

They feel I am too strict with them. If this is the case, when I am strict with them, then what would happen if I became lenient with them?

I know my kids are not geniuses. But consistent study has turned average students into geniuses, it is a proven fact. I only want the best for my children. But they do not understand my feelings and misunderstand me.

Radhika

Counsellor Speaks

Studies form a major bone of contention between parents and children. While parents want their kids glued to their books and tables, children want their own space and freedom to do things their own way.

For Sujata

☐ Within her heart, Sujata knows that her mother means well. Being a rebel and opposing her will not take her anywhere. She and Gopal should show her the results in their exams and sure enough, she will stop coaxing them to study all the time.

☐ Sujata cheated her mother by reading a novel, while showing her as if she was studying. It was likely to break her trust in her children. And this is what precisely had happened.

☐ As a single parent, Sujata's mother feels more responsible towards both of her children. So they should not misjudge her and try to understand her predicament. They should understand her feelings and respect her efforts in doing all that she is doing for them. Once Sujata and Gopal regain her trust and show her results, her stance will loosen and she will give them their required space.

Remote Control

These days our main source of entertainment is television. After a day's hard work, everyone wants to just relax at home and gear up for the next day. In such a scenario, 'who holds the remote…' may turn into a fight for power.

Vineet lives in Nagpur. In their lower middle class family, television is the only source of entertainment. Unlike other households, there is only one television set in his house and everyone has different tastes when it comes to watching programmes.

The members in Bhardwaj family:

Vineet – 19 years old (college student)

Mahendra Bhardwaj – Vineet's father (a government employee)

Sudha Bhardwaj – Vineet's mother (housewife)

Shashank and Shreya – Vineet's twin brother and sister duo (study in class VII)

THE CONFLICT!!!

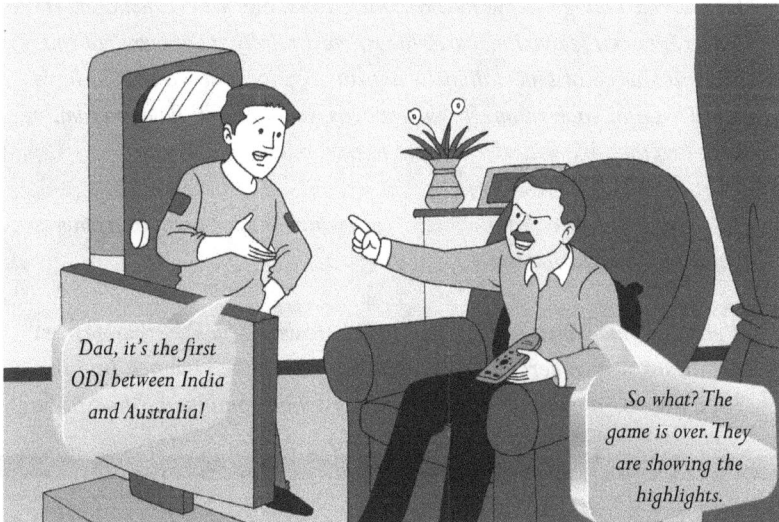

Dad, it's the first ODI between India and Australia!

So what? The game is over. They are showing the highlights.

Diary of Vineet's Father

As children grow older, they become such rebels. These days Vineet is behaving so irrationally. Like yesterday only, he was watching some stupid cricket match on TV when I took the remote from him to watch the election results. He is always watching either some cricket match or some silly English serial which has no truth in it.

I hardly ever sit before TV for long. All I ever watch is News or Discovery or National Geographic channels. I want him also to watch such educational channels so that his general knowledge would improve. But he would only watch fiction.

For him holding remote is like having the magic wand in his hand. If I take it from him he sulks and storms out of the room. This is so unfair. After a whole day's work, I also have the right to relax for a while. Why does he want to make me feel guilty by switching channels and then forcing me to take the remote from him?

Shreya and Shashank never do this. Even he used to abide by me till he entered college. Now he has started making a new demand. He wants his own television set in his room. I totally disapprove of this. TV is a source of entertainment not a necessity that we should have one TV set in each room. If this happens, then we will have no family time together. We will all be glued to our individual TV sets.

It is not as if I own that remote. I only watch one or two programmes before I retire for the night.

Recently, Vineet has started a new trend. He would nick the remote from me during a commercial break and then switch the channel. Initially, I did not say anything, but when this practice continued, I had to be stern and make him understand his limits. I hope he understands that his studies and career are more important than fighting for remote, or his latest demand for a separate T.V. set in his room..

Mahendra

Counsellor Speaks

When life becomes a series of battles over such a trivial thing like remote then it's time to rethink your actions.

For Vineet

☐ Just like Shreya and Shashank, Vineet has been an obedient child who has always walked the path showed by his father. With his new found freedom in college, he has become more assertive and has started putting demands before his father. But these demands are not reasonable. He should not follow them stubbornly.

☐ His father is right in not compromising family time with television. Children tend to go overboard if they are not checked. So not having another television set in Vineet's room is a not such a bad idea.

☐ He can occasionally watch a few programmes of his parent's choice rather than stomping out of the room.

Set Me Free

Everyone likes to live like a free bird. But there is a thin line between living a free life and living a frivolous life. If we flaunt the norms of the society, ignore our duties and live selfishly then it is wrong.

Pranav lives in Panipat. He has a loving family. His sister Pragati loves him very much and tries to protect him whenever required. But Pranav does not come upto everyone's expectations. He seem to have gone off his rockers due to the failures that have led to his frustration.

Let's meet Pranav and his family:

Pranav – 19 years old (repeating class XII)
Pragati – 19 years old twin of Pranav (in college)
Charanjit Singh – Father (owner of a banquet hall)
Shalini Singh – Mother (housewife)
Pragya and Puja – Elder sisters (both married)
Dada and Dadi – Grandfather and Grandmother

THE CONFLICT!!!

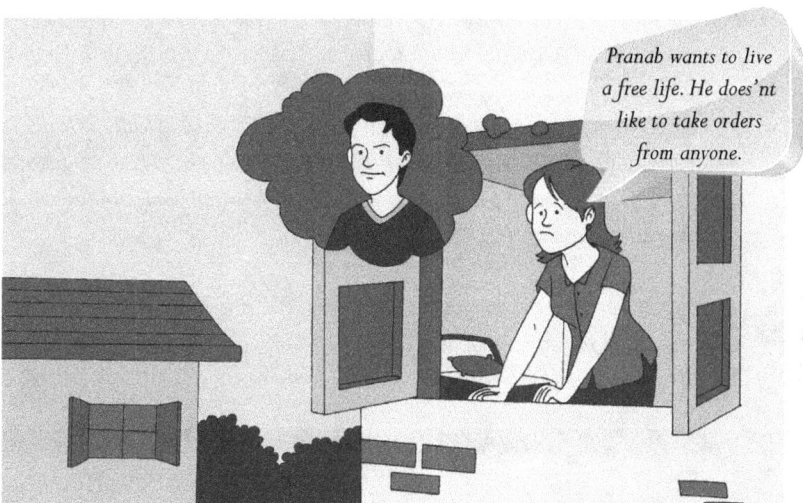

Pranab wants to live a free life. He does'nt like to take orders from anyone.

Diary of Pranav and Pragati's Father

I am on my way home. My work finished last night, but I could get a seat in the morning train.

The atmosphere at home is so stressful that I do not like to spend the weekends there. Pranav has become so rebellious that he cannot take anything I say in the right sense.

He thinks I am standing in the way of his freedom. This began last year when I refused to buy him a bike. That was the first time; he showed his resentment towards me.

Within a moment, he forgot all the love and gifts I showered on him. He thinks that going to disco, malls or movie halls with his friends is a sign of his so-called freedom. This itself shows the immaturity of thoughts.

He flunked once in XII and blames me for this catastrophe. He says that I denied him freedom so he failed. What rubbish! He is not living in a prison, but in a family. Every family has its rules and regulations. It is the duty of every member to follow them. This is how you learn to be social and be accepted in the society.

His single-track mind and his stubborn nature has forced him to think irrationally. He feels that we treat him like a puppet which is definitely not true. If loving your son and expecting him to obey your bidding is considered to be puppetry then so be it.

Pranav is free to take every decision in his life. It is only things which are not good for him, that are denied to him. If he had cleared his boards last year, I was planning to buy him the bike despite protests from his mother and my parents. But he failed me by being adamant and not understanding the actual need of the hour. It was not the bike or his freedom, it was his studies that were so important.

I do not wish to deny him his space and freedom, provided he shows some responsibility. For that he needs maturity which comes with wisdom and stability. His twin sister, Pragati is so much more grounded. I wish he takes some inspiration from her and take his career seriously, not just his freedom and space about which he keeps harping about.

Charanjit Singh

Counsellor Speaks

Today's teenagers are very sensitive. They feel strongly about their surroundings, people and actions.

For Pranav

☐ Pranav accuses his father of being heartless. He feels that his father steals his freedom by not allowing him to have a bike or to go out on his own. But that is not true. His father is only concerned about him. He only has his welfare in his heart.

☐ Pranav should understand that by turning into a rebel he is only harming himself and no one else. If he wants to put in some demands before his father then he should make himself worthy of it. Remember, duties and rights go hand in hand.

What Do I Care!

Sharing and caring are part of a family. Life becomes much more enjoyable when you know there is someone who cares.

Amitav lives in Gurgaon. His family is affluent and they lead a rich lifestyle. However, at times, Amitav misses the love and affection of a loving family despite all the money his parents give him.

Let's meet the Mittal family:

Amitav – 13 years old (student of class VII)

Ranjan Mittal – Amitav's father (successful businessman)

Saroj – Amitav's mother (housewife and socialite)

THE CONFLICT!!!

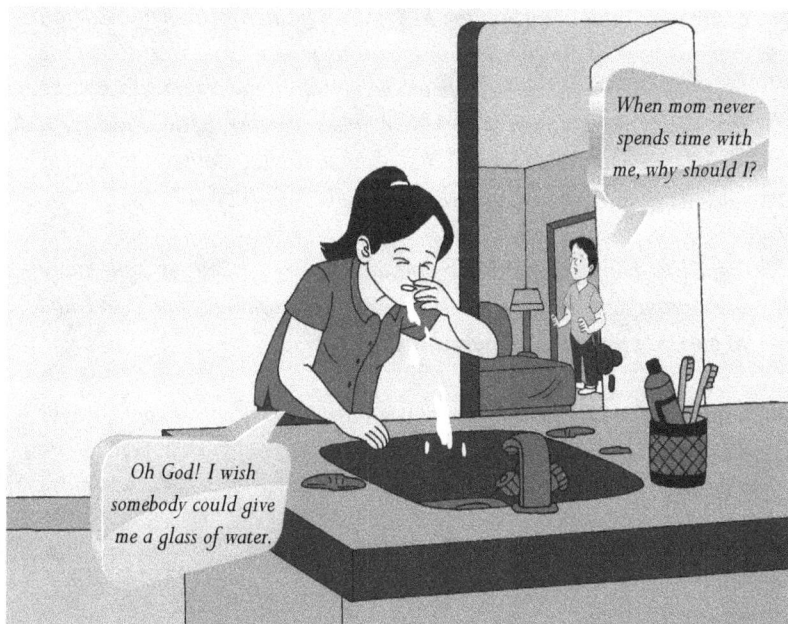

Diary of Amitav's Mother

Sunday , June 2, nightfall

What a strange life I am leading. I have a family yet I have no one to talk to. Ranjan is away most of the time. He is hardly ever at home. Amitav is busy with his school, friends and tuitions.

Last month when I fell ill, there was no one to look after me. I lay in bed the whole day. Ranjan was, as usual, not at home and Amitav deliberately went away to his friend's house leaving me alone. I cried the whole day, but who was there to see my tears. I remembered the good old times when Amitav was small and Ranjan was around. We were a small happy family.

I used to devote all my time to Amitav then. Sometimes, I even neglected Ranjan due to this, but I was sure that he would understand. I did not realise that Ranjan was moving away from us. He started having an affair with his secretary for which he blamed my negligence of him. It shattered me but I had to make a compromise for the sake of my son. I did not want him to grow up in a broken family. Ranjan kept his part of bargain and provided us with all luxuries except for his time and love. I tried to immerse myself in my social life. On the face of it, everything seems okay. Within my heart, I still crave for a complete loving family which we once were. But as they say, past is buried in the sands, what we have in hand is the present.

That day lying on my bed alone and sick, I wished my son would understand that I needed a diversion to maintain my sanity, so I had to immerse myself in my social life.

I know he must be wondering at times why his parents do not care for him like parents of other children do. How can I make him understand that his father has deserted me for another woman? He has made another home with her. He comes here just for formality. But I cannot tell him all this. He is too young to understand such complexities of relationships. So till then, I better keep it under wrap and let things be as they are.

Yesterday, he was looking so ill, but I had some prior commitments so I had to leave him. But before going, I made sure that the maid was there to look after him. Not like that day, when I was in bed the whole day with no one to give me even a glass of water.

Saroj

Counsellor Speaks

Sometimes, what we see is not entirely true. There may be hidden facts behind it which unfold before us when the time is appropriate.

For Amitav

❏ Amitav is at such a stage when he needs both his parents. He does not know the trouble brewing between his parents. But he has an inclination as he heard some gossips from his friend. So he may try to empathise with his mother and instead of trying to settle scores with her, he should be good to her.

❏ Amitav may directly talk to his mother and make her understand how he feels about her detached behaviour towards him. Due to lack of communication, a gap has been created between the relationships. This may be filled by a healthy, heart-to-heart talk.

Attitude Problem

The modern generation or gen Y, as they are called, is quite straightforward. They speak their mind and do not hesitate in making their thoughts vocal.

Sanyukta lives in Delhi. She is a headstrong girl. But sometimes, her stubborn attitude crosses the limits and upsets her parents. Let's meet the Saxena family.

There are four members in the Saxena family:

Sanyukta – 19 years old (Doing first year in college)

Sanjay Saxena – Sanyukta's father (a government employee)

Vandana Saxena – Sanyukta's mother (housewife)

Sanjeev – Sanyukta's brother (an MBA student)

THE CONFLICT!!!

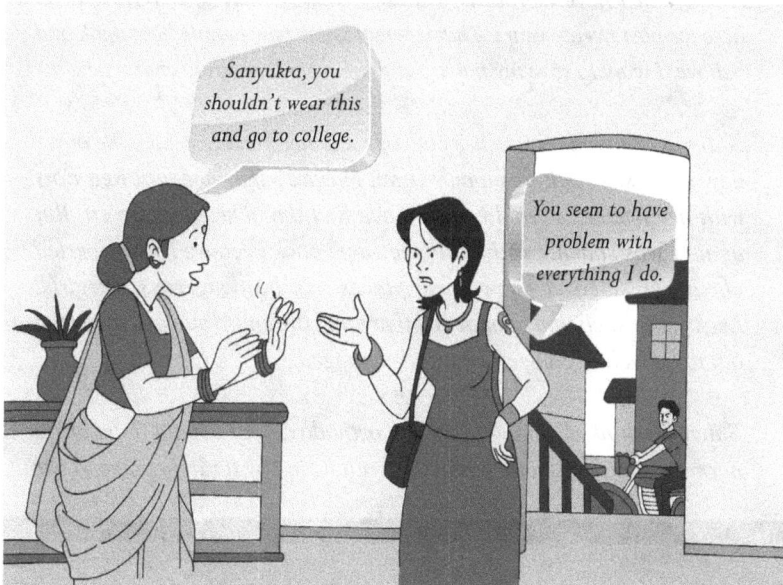

Diary of Sanyukta's Mother

Today was another of those days when Sanyukta and I were at loggerhead. She was going to college in that new spaghetti top which she bought despite my refusal. It was outrageous. Above all, she was going pillion riding with that boy Ronit who looks like a goon.

I wonder where I have gone wrong in my upbringing that this girl always speaks to me so rudely. She has no respect for me, my views and even my orders. She only listens to her father. She has now started treating me as her sworn enemy. She has to defy whatever I tell her without any consideration for good or bad.

She does not realise that what I say is for her own good. My restrictions are only there to keep her safe. Our society is not so advanced even today that she could adopt such outrageously liberal lifestyle.

Sanyukta thinks I hail from a village and I am an old-fashioned. All this is true, but I have learnt the ways of this metro city after having lived here for past twenty years. That is why I know how people here think and behave. I want to save my naïve daughter from the unruly characters.

At times, I do appreciate her courage and her sincerity. Like the other day, when she went to support Anna Hazare's movement at Red Fort with her friends, I would never have had the courage to do so. But again I was shaking within till she came back because I was worried about her safety. I know these places can be dangerous for girls. Luckily, no such thing happened there and the entire movement turned out to be well-organised and well-managed.

Sanyukta thinks I am outdated and orthodox, but I am not. I am just a normal protective mother who does not want any harm to come to her daughter. I am not even trying to possess her. I simply feel it is my duty to show her the right path since she is so young and naïve.

I do not expect much from her except that she shows some respect to her elders and that includes me. I have given birth to her and it hurts when she talks to me so rudely.

Vandana

Counsellor Speaks

In our country, as technology has taken a big leap, so has the culture. The soft-spoken manner of yesteryears is gone and a straightforward approach has taken over.

For Sanyukta

☐ Sanyukta has taken the role of the youth with a zest, but she is going a bit too far. She must understand that there is difference between being straightforward and being rude. She must keep in mind that it is her mother whom she snubs. Education and freedom does not give you the right to reprimand your loved ones.

☐ If Sanyukta mellows down, shows respect to her mother and does not try to act like a rebel by defying the norms set by her mother, then she will find that she has found her best friend in her mother.

9

Dating Blues

Dating is not a new concept in our society now, yet it evokes mixed feelings in parents. Some fear it, some dread it, some simply abhor it. But one thing is sure, they cannot ignore it.

Rachna lives in Kanpur. She is a modern girl who believes that friendship between girls and boys is normal. However, her parents think otherwise. Let's meet Rachna's parents and see what they think about it.

There are four members in Rachna's family:

Rachna – 15-years old teenager (studying in class XI)
Ritu – Rachna's mother (a school teacher)
Raman Chaturvedi – Rachna's father (a police inspector)
Richa – Rachna's sister (recently married)

THE CONFLICT!!!

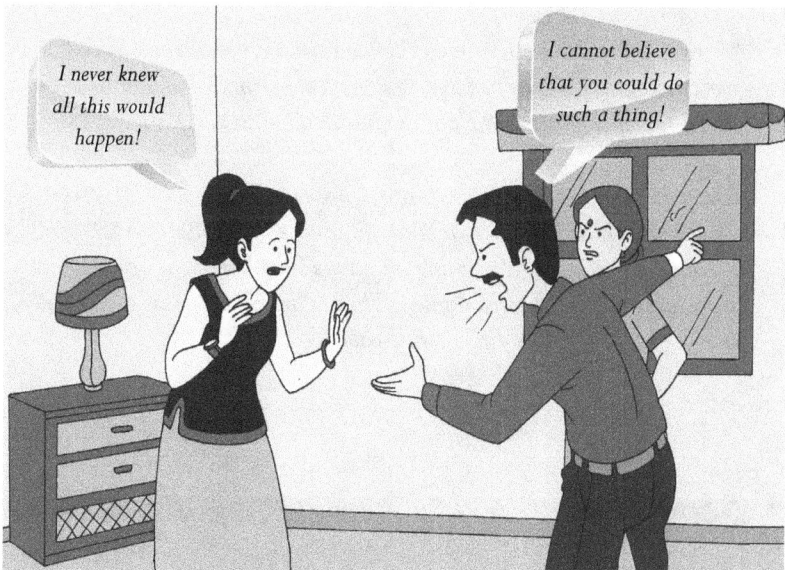

Diary of Rachna's Father

Saturday , October 14, nightfall

Rachna is in her room. After her mother slapped her, she went into her room and locked it. The events of the day unfolded in such a manner, that I felt humiliated and was at a loss of words.

I have always given enough freedom to Rachna, then why did she break my trust? She should have told us before going.

I got the shock of my life when Kadir told me about this incident. Although he was quite calm about it and advised me not to lose my cool. Even I am aware of this police drive which catches couples even if they are just sitting under a tree in a park. They have to show the numbers and today my daughter would have become one of those numbers if Kadir had not called me in time.

I dread to think of what would have happened if any journalist had taken her picture and published in his newspaper for cheap publicity. All these possibilities shunted in my mind and got me really angry.

There could have been many other unfortunate incidences, such as eve teasing by other roadside boys when Rachna and Robin were sitting under the tree in the garden lost in their chat.

I wonder where did we go wrong? I am not so orthodox. If I were, I would not have sent her to study in a co-educational school. Why couldn't she tell us before going on a date? I would have warned her, or at least put some sense in her. What is the point in having liberal views if your own kids do not trust you?

This is a drawback not only in my daughter, but almost 90 per cent of the present day youngsters do not confide in their parents or elders and think that they are always right landing into unnecessary problems created by their own ignorance and wrong decisions.

Raman Chaturvedi

Counsellor Speaks

Life is not always a bed of roses. Sometimes situation becomes so tricky that it requires clever handling of the matter.

For Rachna

❏ Rachna should have confided in her parents before going out with a boy on date. This way, she would have been saved from the embarrassment of humiliation in the police station.

❏ Instead of considering her parents as strict, orthodox people, Rachna should learn to share her feelings and views with them. This may seem useless initially, but slowly it will help her build up a good rapport with her parents

10

Gymming

Being health conscious is good but losing weight on account of food phobia is not healthy.

Let us meet Sadhika who had to face such a problem. Sadhika got carried away by the new fad of being size zero and went on crash dieting. This adversely affected her health. Now she is in a quandary.

Let's meet Sadhika and her family:

Sadhika– 19 years old college student

Sonu – Sadhika's mother, a dietician

Jiten Mansukhani – Sadhika's father, garment exporter

Sujit – Sadhika's 15-year-old brother

THE CONFLICT!!!

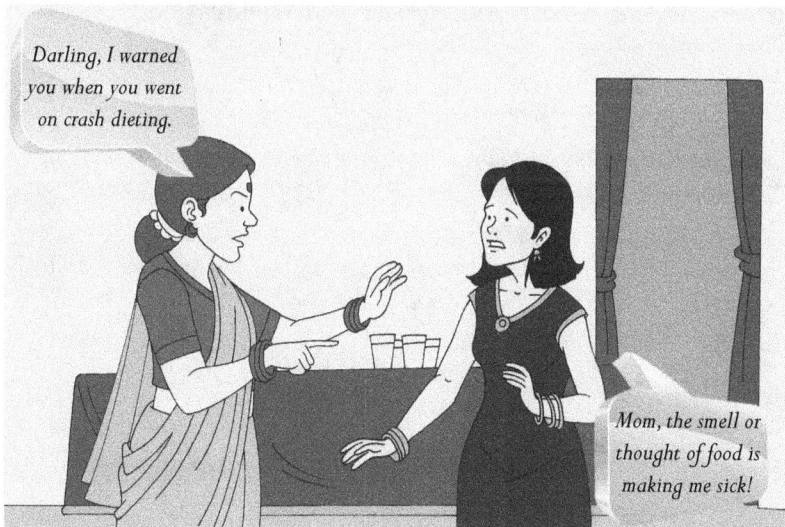

Darling, I warned you when you went on crash dieting.

Mom, the smell or thought of food is making me sick!

Diary of Sadhika's Mother

Saturday, August 19, nightfall

Today was Sadhika's birthday. She had planned this birthday party for a long time. I made so many dishes. But when the party started, Sadhika could not eat anything.

I have been observing her for some time. She has always been plump. After she came to college, she wanted to lose weight and then she got into crash diet. Being a dietician, I know this is not good for health. I tried to warn her. I even prepared a diet chart for her. But like other teenagers, she had no patience. In her hurry to lose weight quickly, she stopped eating altogether.

Today, she has lost the kilos, but at the cost of her health. She cannot enjoy any party, she cannot digest even the simple foods easily. She is popping pills almost every other day. She also suffers from frequent stomach aches and dysentery.

I thought, today she would enjoy, but she had the same bout of sickness again. Sadhika ate lesser than what girls of her age usually eat and that too, after an hour or so, vomitted it all feeling giddy and unwell.

Her friends were worried as she lay still on her bed and the whole party was spoilt. She felt so weak and sick that she couldn't even go to the college, the next day. I am so worried about her but what to do and how?

When I try to talk to her, she feels guilty for what she has done to herself and she just shuts herself in her shell. She refuses to see our family doctor either.

Sadhika blames me for making her put on so much weight. But this is unfair. If she gorges on junk food with her friends, while I am away at work, then how can she blame me for her putting on weight? Whatever genes she has got are not in anyone's hands. Why blame us for that! These same genes have given her a brain which made her a topper in her class, she never blames or credits the genes for that!

Sonu

Counsellor Speaks

Anorexia nervosa is a disease in which the person is afraid of eating. This aversion to food gets instilled in the mind of the person who is dieting for a long time.

For Sadhika

❏ Sadhika's mother tried to warn her against crash dieting, but she would not listen. Now it is wrong of her to blame her mother for not warning her.

❏ Even now it's not too late. Sadhika should listen to her mother and do as she tells her and gain her health back.

❏ Sadhika should understand that being thin and healthy is different from being thin and weak. With the help of her family doctor and her mother, she should learn to eat healthy food.

Mobile Mania

11

There was a time when telephone was a luxury. Today mobile phones have entered the market and they have become a necessity of life.

Shambhavi lives in Hyderabad. As a sign of affluence and modernisation, each one in her family owns a mobile. If the mobile has been considered an important tool for communication, then the family takes it literally and they are on their respective mobiles most of the time. So much so that conversation among themselves has dwindled to monosyllables.

Let's meet Shambhavi and her family:

Shambhavi – daughter (18-year-old college student)
Malti – mother (a boutique owner)
Ravi Prasad – father (import-export business)
Arjun – Shambhavi's 16-year-old brother

THE CONFLICT!!!

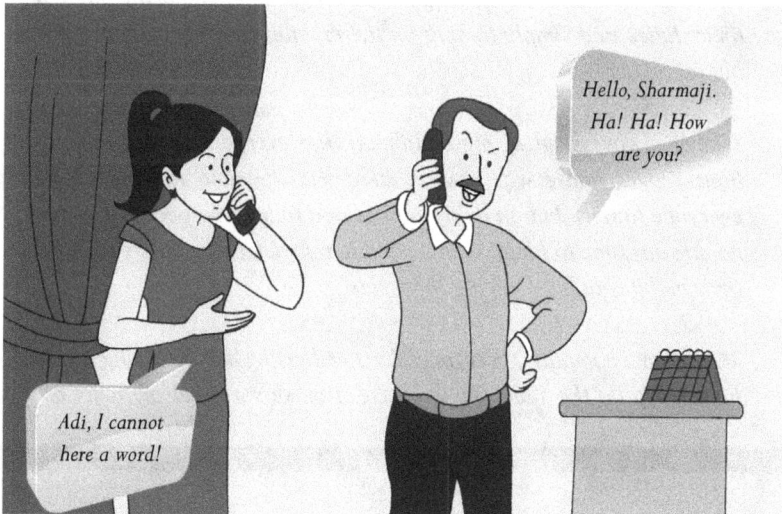

Diary of Shambhavi's Father

Friday, February 12, nightfall

I live in a weird household, where everyone is on their own. I curse the day when we decided to buy four sets of mobile – one for each of us. Today, we hardly converse with each other. There is always someone or the other on their mobile, and we hardly ever get any family time together. I tried to make rules like switching off the mobile during dinner or when we are talking to each other, but it did not work out. Every call is important and no one is willing to sacrifice their independence.

Today I got so angry with this thing that I shouted at Shambhavi. Actually, I had been watching TV waiting for Malti to serve the dinner. But she was busy talking to her client. Shambhavi and Arjun were as usual busy on their own mobiles. In the meantime, my mobile also rang and I started talking to my friend. When I finished, I looked around to find no change in the scenario. This really enraged me and scolded whoever came in front of me.

I feel sorry for taking out my anger on Shambhavi. I did not want to single her out when I was angry with everyone for ignoring me and their duties and simply talking on the mobile. But it somehow came out all on her.

I have always seen in my childhood that everyone would talk for hours. Ours house was always filled with fun and laughter. Here everyone laughs, but on their mobiles and to their respective friends, no one has time to laugh with each other. I wish they could switch off their mobiles at least during the meals.

Whenever I complain, everyone starts criticising me, including Malti, that I also do the same. In any case, I make sure that my calls are short. But it is important for my overseas business because of the time difference. There is no such restriction for the rest of the family. But they would prefer to compete with me and just stick to their own mobiles. Most of the times, I ignore it but at times, I get so fed up that I just let off all the steam.

Ravi Prasad

Counsellor Speaks

Mobiles may be a boon, but there is a dark side too. For those, who value their time with the family, the mobile may prove to be a hamper.

For Shambhavi

☐ Shambhavi should not doubt her father's intentions when he wants the members of his family to switch off their mobile phones and enjoy a meal together.

☐ Shambhavi was angry with her family because of whom her friend could not ask her for a date. But she must understand that if he really wanted to take her out he would ask her later.

12

Tag Along

Parents and children together make a family. Till the children are small, the entire family goes together to each and every function. But once these kids enter their teens, they begin to exercise their likes and dislikes.

Abhijit's parents believe that they should always be seen as a family whether it is a marriage function or a party. They want their children to know their roots and relatives. But in this quest, they go a little overboard ignoring the urgencies and emergencies of children which may bind them from time to time.

Let's meet Abhijit and his family:

Abhijit – 16 years old (student of class X)

Rajendra Vajpayee – Abhijit's father (government job)

Sonika– Abhijit's mother (housewife)

Shikha – Abhijit's 13-year-old sister (student of class VIII)

THE CONFLICT!!!

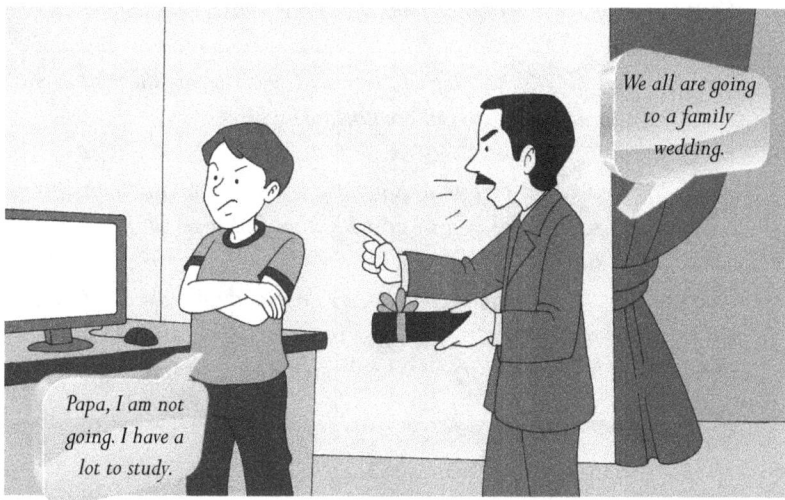

We all are going to a family wedding.

Papa, I am not going. I have a lot to study.

Diary of Abhijit's Mother

It was the first time that I went for a wedding without Abhijit. As a rule, we always go out together as a family. There are many reasons for doing this.

First of all, we do not like to leave children alone at home. So the best option is to take them along. Even if they have an exam the next day, I make sure that they complete their studies and take some time out for the function.

Secondly, it is Rajendra's deep-rooted belief that children will only learn of their lineage if they go out and meet friends and relatives with their parents. He is a very socialising sort of person and he wants his children also to follow in his footsteps.

In any case, it is fun to go out when children are with us. In the hustle bustle of daily life, where is the time for different outings? These functions provide such opportunities when we can go together and spend some quality time with each other.

Abhijit and Shikha have sometimes given this signal that they are no more interested in going to such parties as they have their own group. But I feel they should accompany us (not tag along as the children refer to it) so long as we are all comfortable with it.

However, at times, I feel that Rajendra goes overboard with this ideology and forces children to go with him. But then we have also missed many such functions when children have their exams. In such times, we always skipped the parties. As an exception, last month we had to go to a marriage of a very close relative despite Abhijit's exam. Since they insisted that everyone should come, all of us had to go. But we had told him weeks before to prepare for his exam still he did not do very well in his exam and he blamed it on us.

We have never stopped Abhijit and Shikha from doing what they like to do, why do they then make such a fuss, if we ask them to accompany us once in a while?

Sonika

Counsellor Speaks

There is a clear difference in opinion between two generations. Both are right in their own thinking, so it is better to come to an agreement by taking a middle path.

For Abhijit

☐ Abhijit should understand that his parents are trying to teach them how to socialise and at the same time introducing him to his family. Their intention is genuine and he should appreciate it.

☐ His parents do not seem to be going to parties every day so he can manage to accompany them whenever they go. He should not feel that he is a tag along with his parents because children are an integral part of family, not tag-alongs.

☐ Abhijit too understands that his parents mostly keep his schedule in mind and it was only once that they forced him to go for a party during exam. He feels that due to this distraction, he got bad grades in exam. He may have a frank talk with his parents so that such a thing never happens again.

13

My Friends...Your Friends

We all like to spend time with our friends. But when the parents try to mingle with the friends of their children, then it may not be to the liking of all.

Let's meet Saumya's family. She lives in Indore. She belongs to an upper middle class family. Her parents are well educated and modern. Both her mother and father have jobs which keep them occupied from morning till evening. Being an only child of working parents, Saumya spends most of her time with her friends.

Let's meet Saumya and her parents:

Saumya— 18-year-old college student

Ruchika – Saumya's mother, works as a receptionist

Sachin Srivastava – Saumya's father (a government employee)

THE CONFLICT!!!

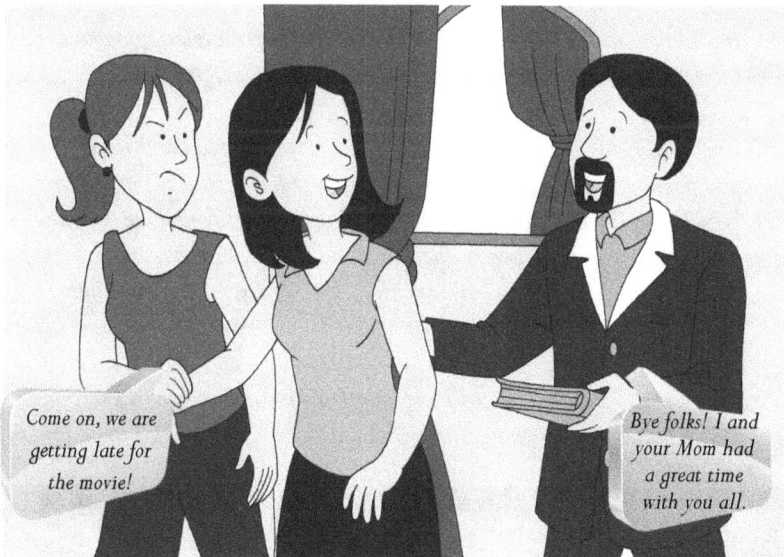

Come on, we are getting late for the movie!

Bye folks! I and your Mom had a great time with you all.

Diary of Saumya's Mother

Sunday , June 19, midnight

Saumya again threw a tantrum today. This is getting out of hand. We have become prisoners in our own home.

Being a single child parents, we learnt all that we could about the younger generation and tried to be friendly parents rather than dominating parents. But it seems all those psychology books and lectures were in vain. However hard we try, our daughter just does not seem to like our friendly attitude.

Whenever her friends come, I try to make them comfortable by talking to them in a friendly manner. Although they all respond in a positive manner, but my own daughter does not like this. She hates to see me or Sachin mingle with her friends.

Earlier, she used to bring her friends often, but now it is very rare that she brings her friends over. In fact, she herself is hardly ever at home. She goes to their homes and praises their parents just to tease us.

It all hurts so much, but I feel helpless. Whenever I tried to make her see reason, she just shuts down and pulls up her defences.

I am a working woman. I do not have so much time to cater to parties and friends. Still I take out time to organise her birthday parties and be with her during those special days. Earlier, she loved it but now she hates my presence in her parties. At times, she even snubs me in front of them which becomes embarrassing for everyone. At such times, I feel like spanking her, but control myself.

I love my daughter and I like to know what kind of group she goes around with. So whenever her friends come over, I sit with them and talk to them. Saumya says that this puts off her friends. She also claims that her friends make fun of our overfriendly nature. I don't know whether I should believe her or not because her friends seem to be quite friendly and comfortable to talk to. They can't be such good actors that they seem something on the face and are something else behind us, or is today's generation double-faced already?

Last year also, she forced me to stay in my room on her birthday. It felt so bad when she asked me to make all the arrangements and go and sit in my room like other parents. I felt as if she had turned me into a maidservant. But for the sake of the peace in the house, I remained quiet. After all it was her birthday and I did not want to spoil her mood. Luckily, Sachin was not there to see all this, otherwise he would surely have scolded Saumya right and left.

I really do not understand the problem in sitting with her friends. If she has her friends' parents as example, I too can quote examples of my friends who have good relations with their children's friends.

Is there something wrong with me, my behaviour or with my daughter? I fail to understand this.

Ruchika

Counsellor Speaks

Teenagers lack maturity of thought and may look at a situation differently from elders. It is the duty of the parents to handle such situations tactfully without hurting the teens.

For Saumya

- ❏ Saumya seems to be suffering from inferiority complex because her mother is more beautiful than her and is much more socialising by nature. Her mother has an idea, but she too feels helpless when Saumya snubs her.

- ❏ Saumya should not compare her parents with the parents of other children. She should be proud that her mother is educated and different from others. This is the fact her friends admire in her mother and she should also accept it gracefully.

- ❏ The parents are not going on outings or be with Saumya and her friends all the time. So it is wrong on part of Saumya to behave in such irrational manner when they try to be friendly with her group.

14

Dressing Spells Doom

Over the years, everyone's dressing style changes. How you dress as a child changes as you turn into a teenager. Similarly, as you grow in life and climb the ladder in social circle, your style of dressing changes accordingly.

Sometimes parents forget that they are not appropriately dressed for their age and this may cause embarrassment for their offsprings.

Let's meet Rishabh who lives with his family in the cosmopolitan city of Mumbai. His father dresses in the modern clothes and at times tries to imitate him. This irks Rishabh as he feels that in this entire exercise, he loses his dignity and respect in the eyes of Rishabh and his friends.

This is the Bhanot family:

Rishabh – 18-years old (college student)
Krishan Bhanot – Rishabh's father (in a private job)
Sushma Bhanot – Rishabh's mother (a beautician)
Ramit – Rishabh's younger brother

THE CONFLICT!!!

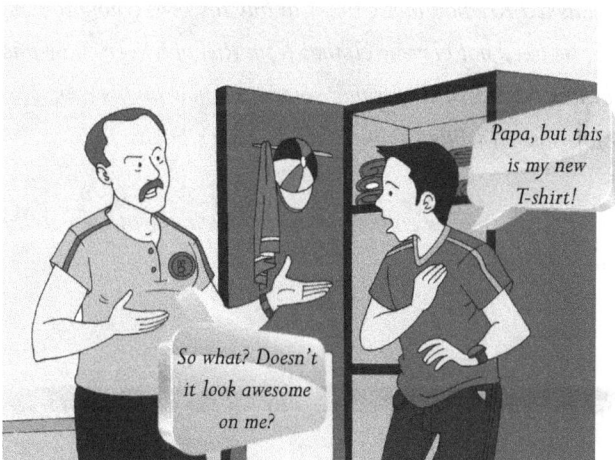

Papa, but this is my new T-shirt!

So what? Doesn't it look awesome on me?

Diary of Rishabh's Mother

Rishabh was very angry today. Krishan again took that new tee of Rishabh which looked so out of character on him. I don't know what is it with Krishan. He seems to have developed some sort of complex. He tries to act and dress much younger than his age. His friends and colleagues laugh on his face, but he just ignores them.

I have tried to make him understand this fact that he should act his age and wear appropriate clothes, but everything seems lost on him.

Although he does not always dress so casually, during office hours, he wears his business suit and looks graceful. It is only when we are out to have some fun like on picnics, parties or outings that he freaks out and wears such outrageous clothes.

I know what irks Rishabh is the way people laugh at Krishan behind his back, but he and I are both helpless.

I have asked Krishan many times to buy his own young looking stuff so that he need not borrow clothes from Rishabh every now and then, but I think he is afraid of trying something new on his own. He wants to enjoy himself while stepping into his son's boots.

None of his friends or colleagues wears such outrageous clothes, but Krishan does not care.

I asked one of my psychologist friend who told me that it was the middle-age syndrome that has caught him which is why he is behaving in such a manner.

Sushma

Counsellor Speaks

Some people do suffer from a kind of complex as they grow old and find their youth slipping away. The love of their family and trust of the family members in them helps them overcome this complex.

For Rishabh

❐ Rishabh's father should understand that he is entering middle age and is no more a young person. He should dress appropriately.

❐ His mother is unable to convince her husband or improve his dressing sense, so she should rope in some good friend of her husband to whom he listens. That person can counsel him.

❐ Instead of getting angry with his father, Rishabh should be patient and empathic towards him. His father seems to be passing the middle-age crisis and he needs help, not criticism. Rishabh may act as his friend and help his father come out of this situation.

15

Career Kit

In today's competitive world, it is a common norm to be ambitious. It is alright if the ambition is towards our own career and life. But when these ambitions cross the line and start influencing the lives of our children, then the trouble brews.

Raman and his family live in Amritsar. Raman's sister did her XII with PCB (physics, chemistry, biology) on the insistence of their father who wanted to be a doctor but could not become one. Unfortunately, Raman's sister could not clear any medical entrance tests and had to satisfy herself with simple bachelor's degree in science. Her dreams of becoming a computer engineer were drowned in her father's ambitions.

Let's meet Raman and his family:

Raman– 16 years old student (just passed X)

Jagdish Malhotra – Raman's father (bank employee)

Suman – Raman's mother (housewife)

Sanjana – Raman's 21-year-old sister (doing B.Sc.)

THE CONFLICT!!!

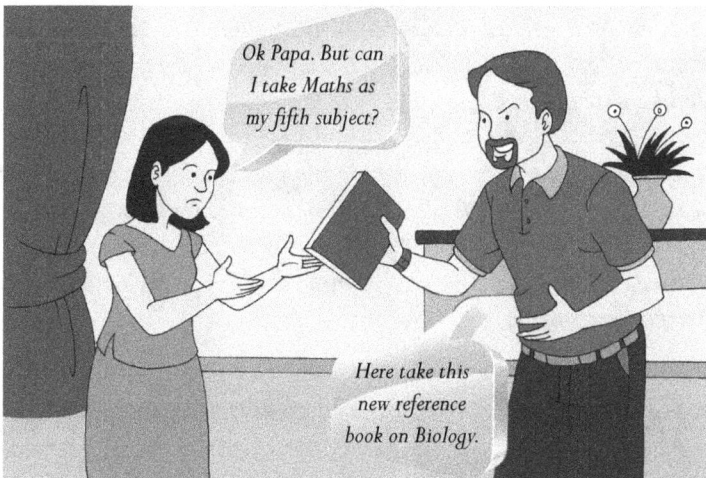

Ok Papa. But can I take Maths as my fifth subject?

Here take this new reference book on Biology.

Diary of Raman's Father

Friday , December 15, evening

I am feeling very low today. Raman's class teacher called me to school today and showed me his results. He failed in three subjects straight. I was aghast. How could I have such dud kids? First Sanjana and now Raman – both have failed me badly.

It was my heart's greatest desire to be a doctor. My father was a small farmer. He always wanted me to follow his footsteps, but I wanted to study and become a doctor. Finally, he gave in and let me study whatever I wanted to. But without a proper coaching, I could not clear the medical entrance exam and ended up becoming a clerk in the bank.

Now I have enough money to pay for my children's coaching fees, but what is the use? None of them is ambitious. I tried to help them in every possible way, but they are not able to study well. They seem to have decided that they must defy me. That is what Raman's results showed today.

I am really disappointed with them. When I told Suman about it, she advised me to let Raman choose the subjects of his choice. I don't know whether it is the right thing to do. Raman is so young. What does he know about his ambition or his future? It is the duty of the parents to guide our children. But it seems whenever I try to guide my children, it backfires.

I am not trying to force my ambitions on my children, but genuinely want them to do well in life. I am willing to pay for it. All that is required of them is to study. And when they fail, if I ever speak of the wasted expenses once in a while, why do they feel so bad about it? Am I not reiterating the truth?

My father was a farmer and he never spared any money for my education. I wish he had, then life would have been so different for me. I do not want my children to live with this regret.

Jagdish Malhotra

Counsellor Speaks

Most of the parents feel that their children are incapable of taking the right decisions about their career, so they try to guide their children. But somewhere along the way, this guidance turns into a command and children begin to feel pressurised under it. To be a true guide for your child, it is important that you do not cross that thin line.

For Raman

❒ Raman's father has the good of his children in his heart. If Raman does not agree with some of his father's views, especially if those views influence his career then he should have the courage and take a stand. He should not spoil his life by simply becoming a meek person and follow his father like a lamb. He must have a heart to heart talk with his father and put his point before him.

❒ Raman's mother may also help him in this matter. Raman should convey to her, his choice of career and his desire to change the subjects in school. She will be able to make his father understand things in a better way.

16

Playing Favourites

In our patriarchal society, the birth of a son is celebrated, while the birth of a daughter is condemned. This discrimination starts from the time of birth and goes on all throughout the life.

Let's meet Arya and her family. Arya lives in Kolkata with her family. Arya studies in a government school, while her younger brother studies in an expensive public school. Arya is good at studies and gets a merit scholarship from her school, still she is not given as many facilities, love and care in her house as her brother is given. Why? Let's read on.

> **This is the Sarkar-family:**
>
> Arya – 14 years old (class IX student of a government school)
> Vimla – Arya's mother (housewife)
> Vijay Sarkar – Arya's father, (a fourth division government employee)
> Siddharth – Arya's 19-year-old brother (class XI student of
>   a public school)

THE CONFLICT!!!

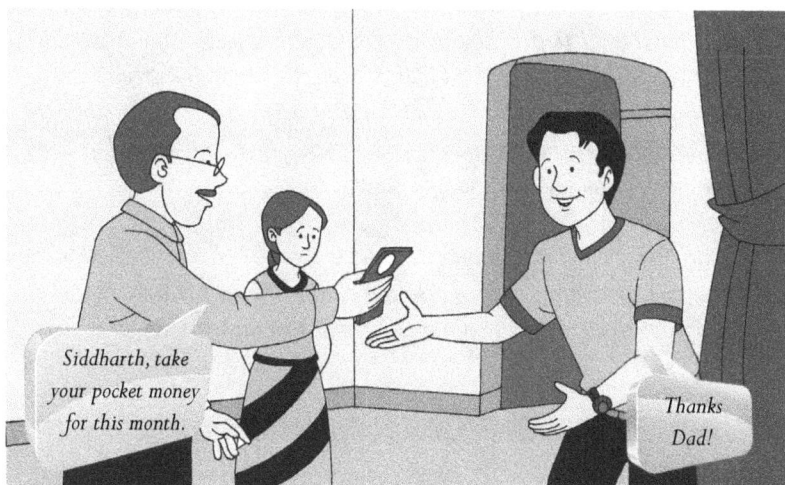

Diary of Arya's Father

Monday, May 20, nightfall

Today Arya and Siddharth's results were declared. As usual, Arya stood first in all the sections, while Siddharth flunked in his class again. The regret of his failing was larger than her passing.

Vimla was almost in tears and I was worried about finance. As it is Siddharth's fees burns such a big hole in my pocket. Now that he has failed, one more year is added to it. Compared to Siddharth, we hardly spend anything on Arya's education. Initially, I wanted both the children to go to the same school but Vimla insisted that Siddharth should be put in an English speaking public school. Her logic was that our son would be looking after us in the old age, so spending money on him is like investing in our future. In a way, she is right also. Even if we get the best education for Arya, she will go to her in-laws' house and they will benefit from her education. As is the norm of the society, I too agreed with Vimla's logic and put Arya in a local government school so that not much money is spent on her. But in my hearts of heart, I sometimes pity my daughter who is such an exceptional student. She has been studying on scholarship, still when it comes to praising her we act such misers.

That day also I felt so bad when Vimla forced me to buy a pair of sports shoes for Siddharth. Later, I came to know that Arya's need for shoes was more than Siddharth's. But it was very late by then. I had already spent my last penny on his shoes. So I could only buy her, shoes after I got my next month's salary.

Vimla always favours Siddharth as he is a son. I also agree with her but at the same time, Arya is also our child. It is not her fault that she is born as a girl. I wish Vimla understands this fact one day and stops discriminating between Siddharth and Arya. This differentiation will result in a rift between the brother and sister in the long run. However, as of now, I decided to keep mum in order to keep peace in my house.

Vijay Sarkar

Counsellor Speaks

Today girls are equal to boys in every field. So it is important that the parents treat them likewise and give them similar love and affection.

For Arya

❏ Arya's feelings are justified as she is the wronged one in this entire scenario. The mindset of our society is such that girls are always considered a burden, whereas the boys are welcomed. Arya's mother is very orthodox in this regard. Since Arya cannot do much to change her views at this moment, she should focus on her goal and work hard towards making her career.

❏ Arya should not feel disheartened if she gets less attention than her brother. She may try to speak to her mother and father and make them see reason. If not her mother, her father is likely to understand. This may not change the situation, but improve it considerably.

17

The Locked Gate

If we rewind for a few years from now, discussing evil was not necessary with our children. Today the time has changed and so has the mindset. With crime rates so high, it is important to equip our children with knowledge of small time evils lurking around us.

Let's meet Suramya who lives in Bareilly with her mother and younger sister. Suramya lost her father three years ago. Her mother got a job in place of her father who was in a government job. As a single mother, it was a big responsibility for her to look after the finances to run the house, provide emotional support to her daughters and arrange for their security at home while she was away at work.

Let's meet Suramya's family:
Suramya – 17 years old (class XI student)
Shalini Bhatnagar – Suramya's mother (government employee)
Sairandhri – 13 years old (class VIII student)

THE CONFLICT!!!

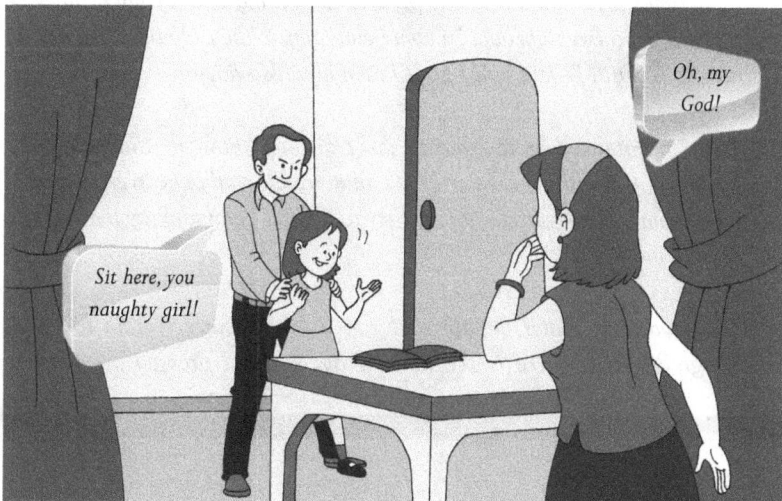

Diary of Suramya's Mother

Sunday, May 28, midnight

Today Suramya came and told me about how Sujit behaved with Sairandhri. I could not believe my ears. Sujit has been such a great support after my husband Amrit passed away. He got everything in order and even helped me get this job. I do not want to lose such a good friend just because my daughter has misinterpreted his action.

But then at the same time, if she is right! Then what do I do? I can't leave my job and sit at home to look after them. I could have called my mother-in-law, but whenever she comes here, she picks up fight with me over the gratuity money of Amrit. She wants that money to be deposited in her name as she claims that he was her son and it is her right over mine over his money. How can I make her understand that this money is neither for her nor for me, I have deposited this money in my daughters' name so that it can be used for their education and marriage. But she is so obsessed with her other son (Amrit's brother) that she wants to give this money to him to start his own business. She has tried all her tactics and when nothing worked, she has stopped coming to this house.

Sometimes, I feel so alone. My parents are no more. Only my brother is there, who lives abroad. In some emergency, the only person I can turn to is Sujit. Where will I go if I turn him also down?

I am so confused as to what to do. I did not show my dilemma to Suramya, but within my heart, I felt shattered. I cannot be everywhere all the time. However much I may try to do, but I cannot play the roles of both mother and father.

Suramya says that I cannot take out a few minutes to talk to my daughters, but where is the time? I am so hard pressed for time.

Commuting to my office takes one and a half hour one side. Then housework, shopping, cooking, washing – all this saps me of all my energy. I am not getting any younger day by day. Age is telling on me and I too want some relaxed moments for myself.

According to Suramya, I should discuss some taboo topics like sex, etc., with her, but I belong to the old school of thought wherein such things were not discussed openly. I still feel hesitant in discussing these things with someone.

I really wish what Suramya is thinking turns out to be just her imagination and nothing untoward happens to my daughters in my absence.

Shalini

Counsellor Speaks

Adolescence is such a delicate stage of life when you are neither an adult nor a child. Care, love and attention bestowed by the parents to their adolescent children can help them face tricky situations of this stage.

For Suramya

☐ Suramya's mother has faced a lot in life so she seems to have got tired with all the blows she had to bear. After living a sheltered life for a long time with her husband, she is finding it difficult to find the ground beneath her feet. In such times, Suramya will have to be brave and take strict stand on her own.

☐ If Suramya is sure of her intuition, she may stop allowing Sujit uncle to enter their house in the absence of her mother. Her mother feels bound to Sujit due to his favours, but Suramya may be practical and act strong. Sujit is doing all this in the disguise of a good friend, but he has his image to protect, so he would not force himself on Suramya or Sairandhri. If she ever finds him going overboard with his overtures, then she may threaten him that she would tell his wife or her mother. It is better to be bold now than sorry later.

☐ Suramya should try to help her mother in household work so that her burden is eased and she has more time to relax and talk to them. This way she might get a patient hearing from her mother.

18

Boiling Over...

Anxiety is not good for anyone. It brings on anger and then we tend to say or do things irrationally.

Let's meet Rahul who lives in Gurgaon. His father is a businessman and quite short-tempered. In his anger, he tends to over-react over things which are otherwise mundane.

This is Rahul's family:

Rahul – 17 years old (student of class XI)

Rima – Rahul's mother (housewife)

Tarun Khandelwal – Rahul's father (businessman)

Simran – Rahul's 12-year-old sister

THE CONFLICT!!!

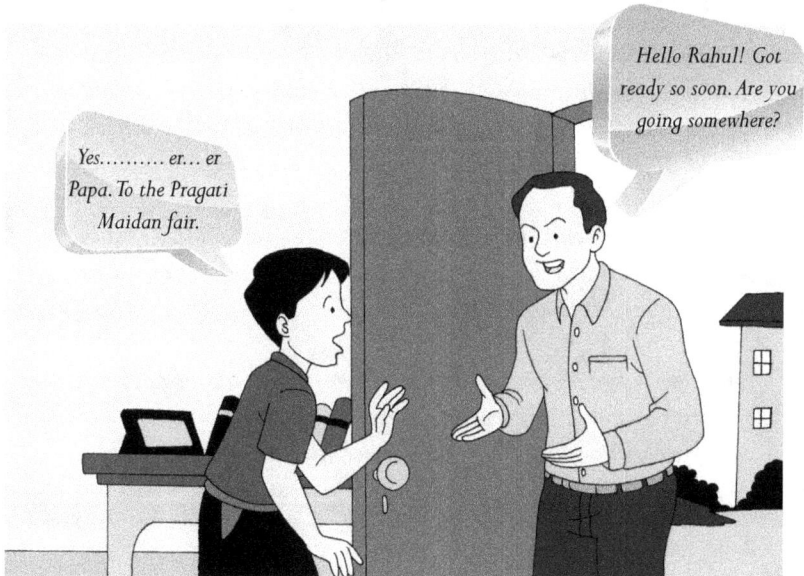

Diary of Rahul's Mother

I had gone to lie down but could not sleep so here I am writing this diary. Tarun's tour ended early and he came back on Sunday morning instead of Monday. And the first thing he saw on returning – Rahul going to IITF with his friends. It gives me shivers when I still think of the confrontation between Rahul and his father.

Luckily, Rahul was so shocked that he could not retaliate. He simply rang up his friends and called off his trip. But I could see from his face that he was so angry and disappointed. After him, it was my chance to bear the brunt of Tarun's anger. He scolded me left and right for even allowing Rahul to go for such a trip at such a tender age. "If this thing happened or that thing happened..." and so on and on he went.

At such times, I feel so restless. I don't know how to make him understand that his son is not a child anymore. One more year in school and he will be going to college. But Tarun's baseless fears cannot be quashed easily.

I have always tried to sympathise with him. My mother-in-law has told me about his troubled childhood when his father was killed in a family feud, his sister was raped and his brother was abducted and killed. She told me that this is why he fears even little things in life.

But he is not a child anymore. He has moved on and lived his life on his own, then why is he hampering the growth of his own child by transmitting his unknown fears to him?

And the worst part is that his fear transforms into anger which he releases on children, especially Rahul. I don't want my son to become as hyper as his father, but I cannot help it. I have seen Rahul getting frustrated with his father's unmindful rantings that I would not be surprised if one day, he too starts acting like Tarun.

Sometimes, when Rahul opens up his heart, he has asked me that why is it that his father always imagines bad things? I wish I could tell him the entire history of his father's life. But he is too raw at present to understand these things. He has a vague idea, but he is not aware of the entire story.

His another grudge is that his father likes to predict things according to his own views. I agree with Rahul. These are Tarun's preconceived notions and fears which make him predict catastrophes in every situation.

I have tried to stop Tarun from making all the decisions for Rahul, but he feels that the only way to protect his son from bad fate and other bad things in life is by keeping him away from all evils that has been happening around him.

Fate has dealt a harsh blow on Tarun which has made him so negative in thinking and deeds. But I don't like him passing on his depression and insecurities to his son like a legacy. I wish I could either change his views or make Rahul understand how much his father has suffered and how that suffering has made him so sour.

Rima

Counsellor Speaks

We all have our shares of good and bad memories. But they should remain only in the past and not influence our present. If they start hampering our and others' life, then they best be forgotten.

For Rahul

- [ ] Rahul should understand that his father is simply extraprotective towards him. Instead of misinterpreting his anger, he should take it in good faith. Till he is in school, Rahul may learn to keep a low profile and not indulge in such activities which enrage his father.

- [ ] Rahul is aware of his father's history. He may sympathise with him. Confrontations, anger or shouting at each other will only ruin their relationship. Luckily, Rahul has no such bad memories which his father has. So it is he who should act maturely and be patient with his father. Sometimes, tables may turn and the *child may actually act as the father.*

19

Nag...Nag...Nag...

Sometimes in our haste to complete work, we tend to push others. This may be acceptable once in a while, but when it stretches to days on end, then it turns into nagging.

Anupama lives in Pune. Her mother is a housewife and obsessed with perfection. Anupama is a well-behaved and diligent child, but sometimes, she gets upset when nagging in the house goes overboard.

Let's meet Anupama and her family:

Anupama – 15 years old (Class IX student)
Anuradha – Anupama's mother (housewife)
Devender Vyas – Anupama's father (accountant)
Avnindra – Anupama's 11-year-old brother

THE CONFLICT!!!

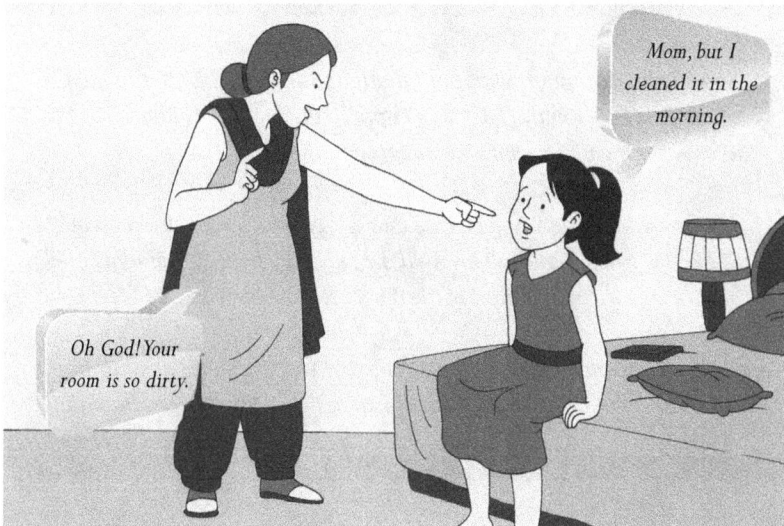

Diary of Anupama's Mother

Sunday, January 16, nightfall

Sundays are always terrible for our household. There is never peace in the house on that day. Either Devender or Anu or Avnindra would throw a tantrum and the whole day is ruined. It is the only day when the whole family is together and I have yet to see a perfect Sunday when everyone relaxes in a spic and span house after a perfect lunch.

But in my house no one is interested in completing their share of work. I work hard in cleaning, dusting, cooking for all of them throughout the week. Then if I ask for some help from them on a Sunday, then why does it irk them so much?

First of all, they would all get up late. Now all the precious morning hours are wasted in sleep. Then they would hover over newspaper and then scatter it all over the place. Their beds are unmade, rooms are dirty and none of them is in mood to have bath on time for lunch. Then they expect me to slog in the kitchen and cook something special.

When I tell them all to clean up or lend a hand in household work, then they call me a nag.

Sometimes, I wonder what am I doing in this unfeeling set of people, whom I call my family. They can't appreciate my efforts and when I try to counsel them, it seems like nagging to them.

I feel as if I am stuck in a vicious circle from which there is no escape. I feel better when I am with my kind, i.e., my kitty friends. But that is only once or twice a month. Rest of the time, I feel as miserable as I feel now.

Even today, all that I wanted Anu to do was do some dusting in the drawing room and then complete her assignments. Since she did not do the dusting properly, I had to do it all over again and due to this the lunch was delayed. When she asked for something to eat, I gave her a fruit and clean her room in the meanwhile till the food was ready. But she did not like it and blew her top.

Anu thinks that I am a perfectionist. But this is not true. Neither am I a perfectionist nor do I expect them to be. I only nag them because they do not seem to take me seriously otherwise. I cannot do everything alone. I need their help which none of them is willing to give without nagging. I know this nagging bit has alienated them to me, but what can I do? When the things go out of hand, I see no other way out. I am like all the other mothers, who love their children, but want them to learn to be independent in life and be proficient in every field.

Anuradha

Counsellor Speaks

Discipline and perfection are important in life, but not to the extent that they start hampering the relationships. Be flexible in your approach and make your home environment comfortable and relaxed and not just plastic perfect.

For Anupama

☐ Anupama thinks that her mother is a nag because she is after her life to complete the tasks she assigns to her. May be if she completed the assigned tasks on time, her mother would be happy and not say anything to her.

☐ Anupama's mother is not a perfectionist, but she wants her children to be perfect in every field. A little cooperation from the children will be helpful now and useful for them later.

☐ Anupama should understand that her mother is not young anymore. May be she is not able to cope up with all the housework. Without getting angry or trying to stay away from her responsibilities, if she lends her full and willing help to her mother, the situation will improve drastically.

Food Row

20

Eating fast food has become a norm of today. Teenagers adopt it more as a fad. This may sometimes lead to difference of opinion between the parents and the teenagers.

Let's meet Supreet who belongs to a middle class family. They hail from interiors of Punjab and now live in Delhi. His father established his business in Delhi and shifted his family here.

This is Supreet's family:

Supreet – 19 years old (college student)
Pinky – Supreet's mother (housewife)
 Gurusharan Singh – Supreet's father (businessman)
Sweety – Supreet's 16-year-old sister

THE CONFLICT!!!

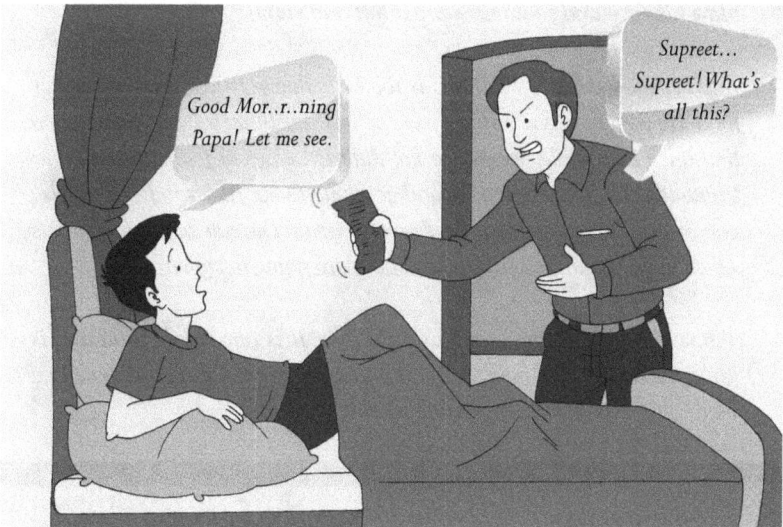

Diary of Supreet's Mother

I do not like showdowns neither does Supreet's father. But sometimes, it becomes inevitable. We are from Punjab, where good and healthy food is always preferred over junk food. We brought up our children with similar traditions.

Earlier, Supreet used to eat home-food happily. But since he entered college, he has started eating out. Initially, it was once in a while, but now it has become a routine. This has affected his health. He has put on so much weight and he has become so lazy. He has lost all his energy.

Within six months, he has become two size larger in his trousers. Sometimes, I wonder if he is eating double the food by eating out and at home as well.

Today, when I discovered the fast food bills from his pocket, it was an eye-opener for us. I was not planning to show those bills to Supreet's father, but he was standing there and he saw them. As expected, he blew his fuse and scolded Supreet left and right.

Supreet's argument is that food is food whether it is fast food or regular food. He is right in a way, but excess of only one thing is bad. I understand that once in a while, we like to eat different types of foods to tickle our tastebuds. But if we overdo it and continue to eat junk food – what else can you call the burgers, pizza, French fries that he eats at fast food joints - then your health and your pocket both are going to suffer.

What we eat at home is a balanced diet. It is our staple food and is good for health. We have never stopped him from eating out once in a while, but this time he has gone too far.

This is a very lame argument that he eats out just because everyone else eats out. You are supposed to live life on your own terms and not on the ones dictated by others.

Pinky

Counsellor Speaks

There are various stages in the life of a teenager which pass away with time. Worrying excessively about them only brings stress to both the sides.

For Supreet

☐ Supreet's mother is right that junk food is not good for health. He must learn to maintain a balance between tickling his taste buds and keeping his health in check.

☐ Supreet should not get angry with his parents when they scold him for doing something behind their back, even if it is only eating out regularly. He must appreciate their concern and be happy that he has such caring parents.

21

Exam Stress

Exams form an integral part of the adolescence. Teenagers spend the best part of their life in school busy with their studies and exams.

Let us meet Garvi who lives in Gorakhpur. She lives with her parents, who have great dreams for her future.

This is Garvi's family:

Garvi – 17 years old (student of class XII)

Ayushi – Garvi's mother (housewife)

Dharmendra Vyas – Garvi's father (an engineer)

Arushi – Garvi's elder sister doing third year B.Sc.

THE CONFLICT!!!

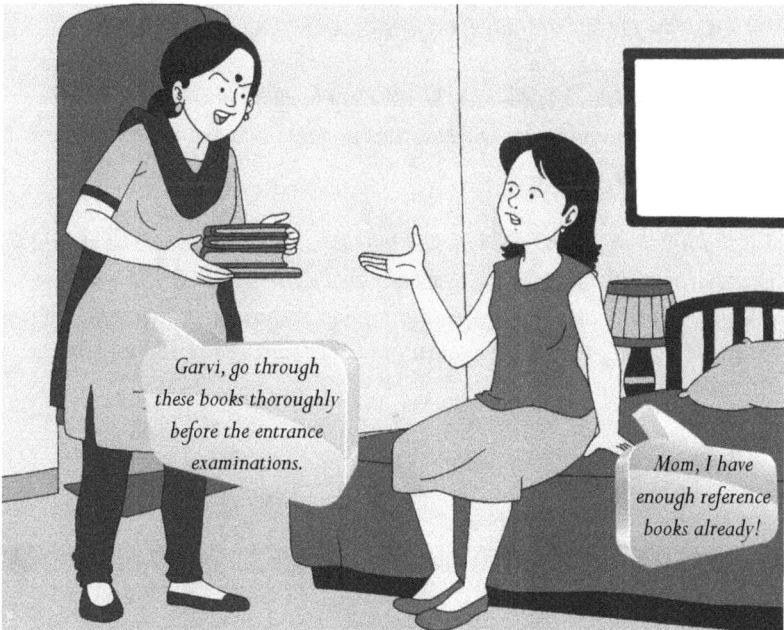

Diary of Garvi's Mother

I don't know what has come over Garvi. She used to be such a good student and now look at her...she looks for any excuse to run away from her studies. First of all, I asked her to take biology in class XI just like Arushi so that she could sit for the pre-medical exams, but she just would not listen to me.

Arushi has been a great disappointment. Even after taking two attempts at pre-medical exams, she could not pass. Now she has no choice, but to do simple B.Sc. and then some other professional course. I am sure, she also did not put her hundred per cent in the preparation, otherwise she would have cleared the entrance exam. I got her so many books, sat with her till late at night, while she studied but to no avail.

Now Garvi is also following her footsteps. She chose to take maths with science and I agreed, though reluctantly. But now that the time has come for her to study hard, she is not willing to work hard.

Why don't these girls understand? They have no brother, their father is a heart patient – they need to stand on their own two feet and secure their future.

Today, when I found Garvi watching that silly movie when she should have been studying for her entrance exam, I saw red. Arushi was also there but instead of telling her sister to go and study, she was enjoying the movie. I controlled myself till the Sharmas went away and then I could not control myself.

I did not want to be so rude and angry, but somehow I lost control.

Garvi thinks I pressurise her so much for studies, but this is the time for her to study. Each moment is precious. She must make full use of each second before her entrance exam.

I have bought so many books for Garvi with the hope that she will study them and benefit from them. But my hopes seem shattered as Garvi is more interested in wasting her time in mundane activities.

I know it is not possible for someone to study all the time. But one should try and use the maximum waking moments so that most part of the syllabus can be covered.

Arushi has proved to be a big disappointment for me and I do not want Garvi to repeat the same mistake. And if Garvi thinks that I am using Arushi as a scapegoat, then she is wrong. I love both my daughters equally, but I am practical enough to admit what and where they have gone wrong.

Ayushi

Counsellor Speaks

In today's competitive world, studying more is never enough. While children need to understand the extent of this competition, parents must also understand that putting extra stress on the children cannot get better results. So it is important to keep their cool and allow the children to be cool too.

For Garvi

☐ Garvi must understand her mother's concern so far as her studies are concerned. Her mother is strict because she wants Garvi to excel in her studies.

☐ Garvi must not judge the equation between her mother and elder sister Arushi by her own standard.

☐ It is true that everyone gets what their fate has in store for them, but it is the duty of humans to make maximum efforts. Garvi cannot ignore this fact and should try to respect her mother for doing so much for her in terms of providing the best facilities to study.

22

It's So Crowded

With changing times, the family system has also been changing. Earlier most of the people lived in joint families, but now the trend has shifted to nuclear families. Whether it is because of migration from rural to urban areas or because of western influence, is difficult to say.

Let's meet Garima who lives in Mumbai. Earlier, she lived with her parents as a nuclear family. Recently, her grandfather died in Patiala and her grandmother had to come to Mumbai to live with them along with her youngest unmarried daughter. Garima finds her small flat very crowded these days.

Let's meet Garima and her family:

Garima — 14 years old (studies in class VIII)

Sangita — Garima's mother (housewife)

Ashok Sahni — Garima's father (employed in a private firm as clerk)

Sanchit — Garima's 11-year-old brother (studies in class V)

Dayawati Sahni — Garima's grandmother

Shalini — Garima's aunt (yet to be married)

THE CONFLICT!!!

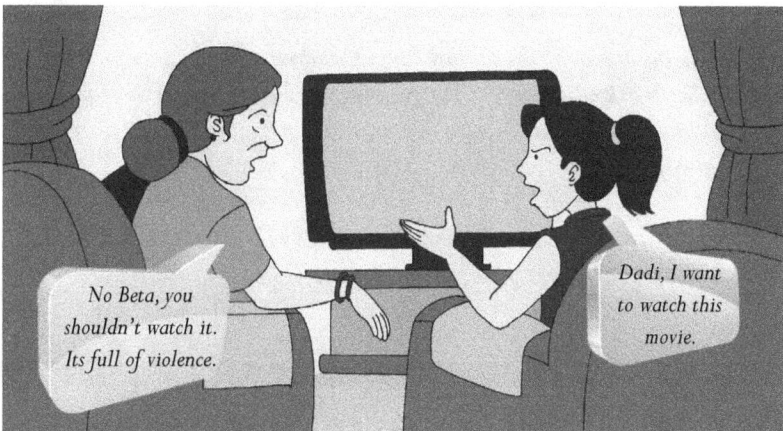

No Beta, you shouldn't watch it. Its full of violence.

Dadi, I want to watch this movie.

Diary of Garima's Mother

Saturday, June 20, midnight

I felt very sorry for Garima today as she came to me to cry her heart out and I could not do anything. I do not blame her as she has not done anything wrong. She was simply watching her movie when Mataji (mother-in-law) suddenly changed the channel. We cannot even tell her not to do such a thing because then she creates such a scene over little issues that it is better to remain silent.

I know Mataji also feels suffocated in this house. She has come from a small city, where life was simple and easy. She is used to living in a big house which she has sold now. Earlier, we all lived together but later when we shifted to Mumbai after Garima was born, she and Pitaji (father-in-law) stayed back in Patiala with Shalini. Now Mataji has now got used to living independently and so have we. In a way, our joint family broke into two nuclear families and now we are all finding it difficult to go back to same joint family routine. My children grew up in the metro culture with an independent way of life. Now all of a sudden, this turn of fate has brought us all together and we are in a fix.

Children are the worst affected as they have lost their room, their studies are suffering and they cannot lead the kind of life they are used to.

T V is on in our house all day long. Children cannot study properly. Kitchen work and other work have also increased. Neither Mataji nor Shalini help me at all. Not that I am complaining, but I would also like to have some time free when I can look after my children.

I know there are many advantages of joint families, but that is if all the members understand their responsibilities.

But at the same time, we cannot ignore the fact that they are our own people and they need us.

Garima has hinted many times that either we should take a bigger house or send her to hostel. I wish I could make her understand that we are not so rich as to be able to afford either of these. Besides, we need to save some money for Shalini's marriage.

The only option left is to ask Ashok to speak to Mataji and settle things amicably because being a daughter-in-law, her orthodox mindset will not allow her to accept any advice I give to her.

Sangita

Counsellor Speaks

After living in a nuclear family for so many years, it becomes difficult to adjust in a joint family. While nuclear family comes with a certain freedom, joint family poses many bonds which seem too binding if relations are not congenial.

For Garima

❏ Garima must understand the situation from the point of view of her grandmother. The circumstances have forced her to come here after leaving her native place. She too must be feeling like an outsider. She must make friends with her not treat her as her rival.

❏ Garima must accept the fact that her parents are not so well off that they could either take a bigger house or send her to hostel. So she may make the best of the situation by befriending her Dadi and Bua. This way she may not find the life so tough.

23

I Am Not Yours

The bond between a child and the parents is special. No one can break that bond. This bond has its roots in the love and affection that both feel for each other.

Does being an adopted child or a biological child have any affects on this bond? Let's meet Mita who is an adopted child. Her parents legally adopted her from an orphanage after ten years of their marriage and showered all their love and affection on her. Being liberal and open-minded, they did not hide this fact from her and on her 18th birthday told her everything. Should Mita feel angry, hurt or obliged?

This is Mita's family:

Mita – 18 years old (studies in class XII)

Manju – Mita's mother (housewife)

Mahendra Nath – Mita's father (businessman)

THE CONFLICT!!!

Mita Beta, we would like to tell you something.

Mom, Dad! What is it?

Diary of Mita's Mother

Tuesday, July 15, midnight

Since I told Mita everything about her adoption, I have been asking myself – have we done something wrong? I feel so disoriented. It is because of the reaction that we got from Mita after she got to know that she is not our biological child.

*We waited for her to grow up so that she could understand our feelings and not take this news otherwise. I still remember that fateful day clearly when doctor had declared that Mahi was unfit to father a child. We thought a lot, consulted more doctors. Some even suggested sperm donation, but I was not ready. In the end we zeroed in on adoption. There was no dearth of wealth in the house; all that it lacked was a little baby to enjoy it. We decided to adopt a child from an orphanage called the **Mother Teresa Home**. When I first saw Mita lying in the cot playing with her big toe, I lost my heart to her and I became desperate to bring her home.*

She was merely two months old when she came to our house. I looked after her, loved her, cuddled her, played with her. In fact, I did everything a mother does to her daughter. Then why would just one word adoption change all that. Mita taught me the meaning of motherhood. She filled our lives. She made me complete. She is the apple of Mahi's eyes. Whatever we have is hers. Then why is she taking it so hard? I never anticipated such reaction from her, otherwise I would never have told her. If we could hide this fact from her for 18 years, we could do it for lifelong.

But Mahi was insistent that we should not keep her in dark. He says there should be no secrets from those whom you truly love. So I gave in and agreed to tell her the truth. Within heart of hearts, I was confident of my upbringing and love for her. I knew she would understand and then forget all about it. But it seems I was wrong. She got so upset that my heart sank on seeing the expression on her face. She wanted to meet her biological parents. But where are they? There was no detail about them in the orphanage records. And in any case, what does it matter now? Is it not enough for her that she is our daughter. We love her and she loves us and that is the only truth that exists for us. Her position in the house is not going to change just because she knows some silly truth which we have known for past 18 years.

Silly girl.

I am sure she will come around soon. I feel sorry for having caused her so much distress, but as Mahi says, we should endure pain with a brave heart if it is for our own good. Mita is our daughter and she has grown up with our values. She will come around soon.

Manju

Counsellor Speaks

Adolescence is a stage when you are neither a child nor an adult. You are not expected to act childish and at the same time, you cannot act mature either.

For Mita

❏ Mita should respect the honesty and sincerity with which her parents have handled the entire situation. They could have kept mum and not told her the truth all her life, but would that not be equal to deceiving her? And what if she got to know of the truth from someone else? So she must respect their noble feelings instead of blaming them.

❏ Mita's quest for search of her biological parents is nothing but her running after a mirage. First of all, she does not even know their names and whereabouts. If by some quirk of fate, she find them, would she ever feel the same for them as she feels for her adoptive parents?

❏ Mita should learn to accept the good things the fate has offered her in a platter. She must remove all misgivings from her mind and learn to count her blessings.

Special Needs

24

It is a misconception that we should treat children with special needs differently. If you ask them you would understand that they too like to be treated as normal.

Let's meet Robin who is hearing impaired. Robin lives in Goa. He has a loving family, but sometimes, he likes to be independent because he feels that he can look after himself.

This is Robin's family:

Robin – 16 years old (studies in class X)

Mary – Robin's mother (housewife)

Joseph Fernandez – Robin's father (shopowner)

Rubaina – Robin's sister (studies in second year college)

THE CONFLICT!!!

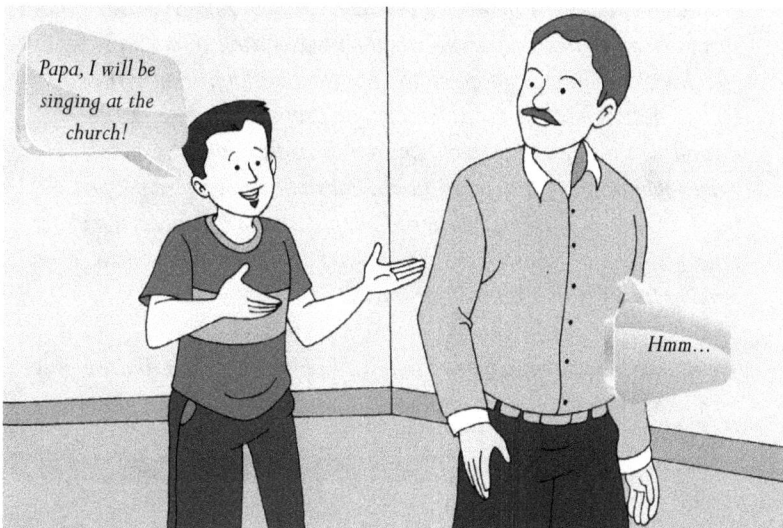

Diary of Robin's Father

Today was a big day for Robin. He has been working hard on his speech coordination and it has paid off. Although he wanted to give us a surprise, but father in the church let us on in his secret. Father seemed quite confident of Robin's ability to sing, but I could not dispel my own apprehensions. This was why when he gave me the news as a surprise in the morning, I could not play along. I was too busy in my own apprehensions. Thank God everything went well.

I have been noticing some changes in Robin recently. He has become more assertive. He wants to be independent and does not like when we try to help him. Like today, when Mary tried to take Robin's hand while crossing the road, he tried to break free. We have always taken care of him because we know he cannot hear the horn and he has never refused. But today, he just did not want anyone's help. This surprised me to see my meek son suddenly being transformed into an independent boy. May be success does this to people. But how can I make him understand that living in this world is not as simple as singing Christmas carols? He has a disability and he will have to face problems because of them. We are there to help him. He should not shrug us away like this. Even when he was sitting in car in front of the church, some people came to congratulate him. I knew that they had come to check, if Robin can speak properly despite his hearing disability. I wanted to protect him from their false praises and did not want them to mock him later. Robin does not know these people, but I know them well. They are wicked people, whom I have seen making fun of others in front of me. Then what is there to stop them from making fun of Robin behind our backs?

We are definitely not ashamed to have Robin as our son. But we only try to save him from this harsh world. He is still young and naïve. I am sure even if I had a normal son, I would have protected him in the same manner.

We do not want to be his ears, we know he is learning to be independent, but we can't leave him alone till he is proficient in facing the world alone. At this moment, he needs our love as well as our help.

Joseph

Counsellor Speaks

Life for a challenged child may seem difficult for us, but it is not always so. God gives his people enough courage to overcome any crisis. So what seems like a handicap to you, may be just a way of life for that person who is born with it. So do not judge others with your own perception. Give your child his independence to follow his dreams.

For Robin

☐ Robin's parents have his welfare on their mind that is why they try to protect him. He should not misunderstand them and return their warmth with love.

☐ Robin should be happy that he has overcome his physical handicap with his efforts, but there are people who think themselves superior to others. So Robin should accept his parents' help till he is old and experienced enough to understand the psyche of such people.

25

Listen to Me

Some people show attention-seeking behaviour. This may stem from some childhood experiences, low esteem or inferiority complex.

Abhishek lives in Jaipur. He is the youngest son of his parents. His eldest brother Abhinav is bright in studies, while the second brother Anuj is a good sportsperson. Abhishek is a mediocre in every field. He is an average student and has no interest in sports. Since he feels inferior to his brothers, being the youngest in the family, he often throws tantrums.

Let's meet Abhishek and his family.

Abhishek – 14 years old (studies in class VIII)
Abhinav – 22 years old (doing MBA)
Anuj – 18 years old (plays cricket at national level)
Aradhana – Abhishek's mother (lecturer)
Dr. Vishwa Mohan Singh – Abhishek's father (Doctor)

THE CONFLICT!!!

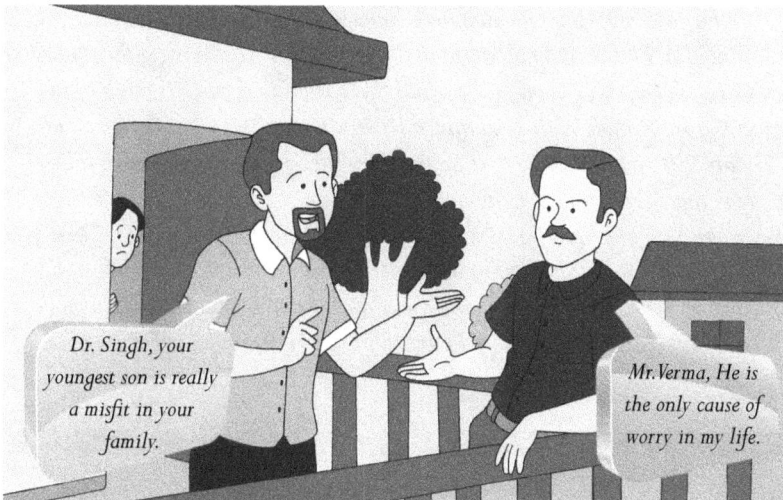

Dr. Singh, your youngest son is really a misfit in your family.

Mr. Verma, He is the only cause of worry in my life.

Diary of Abhishek's Father

Saturday, April 10, midnight

Tonight after dinner, when I was moving towards the balcony along with the Vermas, I heard the door slam. Immediately, I understood that Abhi had heard our talks. I feared another tantrum from him, but luckily the boy kept mum. Normally, when he gets into a bad mood, he throws things around, breaks a few things and generally attracts attention to himself.

I used to be angry with him, but ever since I understood that he does this as attention seeking tactic, I feel sorry for him. I know it is not easy to live in a house, where everyone reminds you how mediocre you are. I am happy for my two elder sons, as they have emerged achievers. But I believe that every individual is an achiever in his own right. The day his calling comes, he will also bloom like a flower.

His behaviour is triggered by the reaction of insensitive people, who just like to interfere in others' life. Like that day, when Aradhana's cousin Suman commented on Abhi's behaviour and suggested that we send him to hostel. I know Abhi is very sensitive, but I wish he learns to keep his emotions in check and stop throwing tantrums.

Who says my Abhi is a mediocre. Last week, I discovered an amazing talent in him which no one in the family has. I was looking for a pen, so I entered his room. He was not there, but a beautiful sketch of our villa in Manali with beautiful hills in the backdrop sat on his study table. It seems he had just finished it. There was a big manila folder on the table. When I opened it, some most beautiful sketches and paintings fell out of it. I kept staring at them for some time. Then I felt as if I was trespassing on someone's property. With a guilt in my heart, I closed the folder and went out of the room. But the memory stayed. His paintings were beautiful. I wanted to tell Dr. Verma about his paintings, but held myself.

No, my talented son needs no introduction. I will talk to him soon about his paintings and if possible, hold a private exhibition for some select audience. But till then, I wish I knew how to keep his frustrations away and curb his attention seeking behaviour.

Abhi feels that we love his brothers more than him, but this is not true. For parents, all their children are alike. We have accepted him with all his faults and virtues. I have never put him down before anyone and would never ever do it.

Vishwa Mohan Singh

Counsellor Speaks

Many children show attention seeking behaviour when they are low on confidence. This habit should be curbed as soon as possible by dealing with the child in gentle, yet firm way.

For Abhishek

☐ Abhishek has a hidden talent which his father has recognised. Abhishek must come out of his cocoon and share his talent and happiness with others.

☐ Abhishek must understand that his parents have never discriminated between him and his brothers. It is his inferiority complex that makes him attempt attention seeking behaviour. He must have faith in his abilities and his parents. The rest will be easy.

Parenting Marvels

Parents form a very special species in this world. On one hand, they seem so strict and on the other hand, they are so lenient that their own child is not able to fathom the extent of their character. But when they are among their own kind, i.e., with other parents, they share a good rapport. The major topic of discussion among parents is invariably their children. For them bringing up children is the most complex, challenging and tricky task in the world. They may conquer Mount Everest, solve tricky algorithm problems and bear any amount of work pressure but when it comes to child rearing, they buckle under the strain and demands of this task. But before you get some weird ideas, I will let you into their cherished secret, they love every bit of parenting.

Let's see what PARENTING is all about –

P – Perseverance

A – Affection

R – Resourcefulness

E – Efficient

N – Nurturing

T – Tactful

I – Insightful

N – Natural

G – Guide

Altering Role of Parents

There exist no simple and straight formulae for parenting. There are no hard and fast rules for a particular response from the parents in any given situation. The way parents deal with their children is a combination of their own experiences, the individual needs of the child and the environment.

The child-parent relationship undergoes change with the time. When the child is born, the parents are filled with joy. They experience joy combined with anxiety as the newborn grows. The dedication and understanding about the needs and wants of the child change their outlook towards life.

As the child grows up, parents derive a lot of satisfaction from their handiwork and this transforms into enormous love they feel for their child. They manage to obtain a super memory and store their child's first words uttered, the first steps taken, the first sentence etc, into it. They indulge and pamper their child and derive immense pleasure and satisfaction from it. Soon the child becomes the apple of their eyes and the centre of their existence.

During the teens, the loving relationship between the child and the parents undergoes a sea change. Confrontation and arguments creep in and form an integral part of their life. While the teenager is not the obeying child anymore, hanging on to each and every command of their parents, the parents are not all that understanding and patient as they used to be.

Organisers

The relationship between parents and children becomes complex when the parents see themselves as the organisers for their children's lives. They try to manage the lives of their children constantly. They love laying the ground rules for them, making sure they follow them and constantly badger them on what to do and what not to do. This arrangement works fine till the children are small, but as they grow up, they start asserting themselves and this is where the tiff begins. Children have their own ways of doing things which may not make sense to their parents. In such cases, the difference of opinion leads to conflicts in the family. Communication is very important for any relationship to survive.

Parenting Styles

Each parent has a different style of parenting depending upon one's individual way of thinking, attitude, upbringing, socio-cultural background, education, career growth and development. In a broader perspective, there are three different parenting styles:

- **My Way**

    'I' or the parent takes all the decisions. Such parents order their children about. They tell their children what to do and what not to do. These type of parents want total obedience from their children in any circumstances. They leave no choice for argument or discussion. This parenting style is good in certain situations where parents are required to be firm and disciplined like not allowing your son to drive a car before 18 years or not letting your daughter go for late night movies.

□ Your Way

'YOU' or the child takes all the decisions. In this type of parenting, parents do not interfere or control their children. They allow their children to take their own decisions and face the consequences, whether good or bad, themselves. These are the parents who believe that this would make the children more confident and they should learn from their own mistakes. This type of parenting has many advantages like children become independent, their decision-making ability improves and they learn through practical experience, but there are some drawbacks too. The children might misuse the freedom given to them. Children being immature may take a wrong decision and then suffer the consequences without any help from the parents.

□ Our Way

'WE' take all the decisions together. Here the stress is not on 'I' or 'You' but it is on 'We". This is a blend of the first and second style of parenting. The problems are sorted out jointly and the decision-making power lies with the children, but the decision is taken after the parents and children sit together and arrive at a solution that is agreeable to both. Sharing is the key word in this style of parenting. This parenting type has been found most appropriate as children are able to learn and perform better and they grow up to be mature humans.

Parental Paranoia

The parents of modern society suffer from an obsessive condition called *panic parenting*. The main feature of this condition is the desire of the parents for their children to excel in every activity – be it studies, sports or dramatics – you name it and they want it. The parents of today are joining the bandwagon of high-speed competition without comprehending the nature and needs of their children and the rat race they are pushing them into.

Panic parenting puts tremendous pressure on the children and sometimes leads to their nervous breakdown. Panic parenting begins from the moment the baby is conceived. The sex of the child is determined by scanning, the meaningful name for the child is searched, sometimes the child is even registered in a good, reputed school before it arrives in this world. When the child is born, his height, weight, speech, gait and other activities are carefully monitored. Then begins the rush and stress of studies in school. From play school to college – there is no end to *parental paranoia*.

In all this if the children grow up with anxieties and out of frustrations get involved in issues like alcohol, drugs, sex and crime, then where is the time to excel? The children may also end up with stress related disorders like palpitation, nervousness, erratic blood pressure, insomnia, loss of appetite, depression, etc.

So the need of the hour is for the parents to take a wakeup call and understand that their child is an individual. They should support their children and guide them with love and affection. They must refrain from exerting undue pressure on children and should not expect them to achieve way beyond their abilities. Instead of goading them, they should act more like a friend, philosopher and guide to their children rather than being a critical, demanding and pushy dictatorial parent. This is bound to lead them to parental success.

Grievances

Parents Talk

Q1. *My son speaks rudely with us. Any type of cajoling or gentle talk does not seem to make him realise his folly. What should I do?*

Ans. First of all, you must analyse your own behaviour and assess if you have ever been rude to him. Most of the times, children like to imitate their parents. They learn habits, good or bad, from their parents. Show him with your actions that you do not like this way of talking and he must amend his ways.

Q2. *My daughter watches TV all the time even at the expense of her studies. Ours is a joint family, so the TV is always on in our house. What should I do?*

Ans. Provide your daughter a room farthest to TV, where she can study in peace. Since you cannot stop others from watching TV, you will have to make your daughter understand the importance of studies. Allot her a specific time during which she should study. In rest of her free time, do not stop her from watching TV, if she wants.

Q3. *Despite my repeated warnings, my 15-year-old son takes my bike and goes for a ride with his friends. I have a touring job so I am out of town most of the time. What should I do?*

Ans. You have only two options – either you rein in your son or sell your bike. Because if your son is caught riding a bike without licence, he may be prosecuted. So take a firm stand. If you are not there, ask your wife to be firm and not hand over the keys of the bike to your son. Gently make him understand that he should wait for a few years till he gets his licence.

Q4. *I am a morning person and I want my children to be up early. But they like to study till late at night and wake up late too. Am I wrong in teaching them some good habits?*

Ans. You are absolutely right that waking up early in the morning keeps you fresh and healthy. If they are so adamant on studying at night, you may ask them to try this new schedule for a few days and see how different they feel and fare in studies. If your children still prefer night time to study than the morning hours then let them be.

Q5. *Ours is a very religious family. We often have havans and kirtans in our house. My daughter who is in class XII gets very irritated because of this. Although we have given her a separate room for study, still she continues to complain as the hustle-bustle of the function disturbs her. What should I do?*

Ans. You may have made all the arrangements you deem fit for your daughter so that she won't get disturbed, but the problem is that she is still getting disturbed. You may try sending her to her friend's house or to a relative's house nearby, where she can study without interference.

Adolescents Talk

Q1. *I feel disillusioned when my parents compare me with my friends when it comes to studies. What should I do to stop them from doing this?*

Ans. Sit down with your parents and tell them frankly that you do not like to be compared with others. Tell them that every person is an individual and one cannot be compared to another. Ask them how they would feel if you were to compare them with your friends' parents.

Q2. *I want to play video games in my free times, but my parents insist on my going out and play outdoor games. Whenever they see me playing games on computers, they just blow their fuse. What should I do?*

Ans. Your parents are right in telling you to go out and play in fresh air. Video games do not provide you exercise in any form. Restrict your video gaming activities to a limited time period and balance your studies, outdoor games and video games giving appropriate weightage to each according to the advantages you derive from them.

Q3. *My father uses swear words even in the house, but whenever I use one he scolds me. Why these double standards?*

Ans. Talk to your mother and include her in your problem. Ask her to make your father understand that he too should not use such words. Children learn what parents do before them. If he will stop using swear words, chances are that you will also soon get out of this bad habit. He must understand that he can only stop you from doing something by being a role model himself.

Q4. *My parents insist that I should read newspapers, news digest and other magazines like "Competition Success Review", while I like easy reading books and stories. Is he right or am I right?*

Ans. A reader has no limits on reading. If you are a good reader, you would devour newspapers, news digest, etc., with equal fervour as you would do with books and fiction. Your parents are right in showing you the right direction because in today's competitive world, it is very important to remain updated on current affairs. While fiction tickles our imagination, news magazines provide us a plethora of information. Grab both and expand your horizon.

Q5. *My parents balk at the mention of group studies. Being an only child, they keep a hawk-eye on me and do not allow me to study in groups. They think that I will waste my time with my friends.*

Ans. Group study is not bad if you do it sincerely. In fact, it is rather useful because you get to learn more with many different minds working together. But if you take group study as an excuse to be able to spend time with your friends, then it holds no value. Now it is upto you how you study in a group. Keep one thing in mind that your parents can judge your level of study with your performance in class. So if you do genuine group study, then talk to your parents and make them understand the importance of group study for you. Ask them to give you a chance and then see your results. In most likelihood, your parents will understand your point of view and allow you to study in a group.

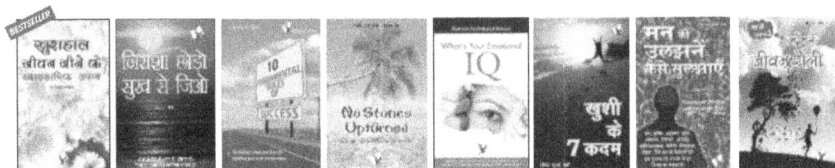

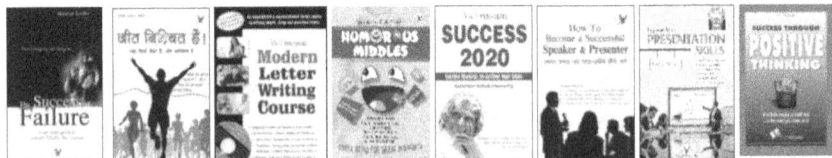

Also Available
in Hindi

Also Available
in Hindi

Also Available
in Kannada, Tamil

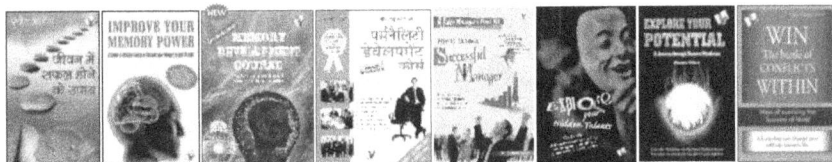

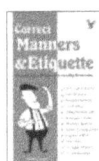

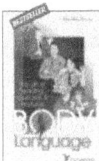

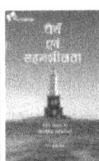

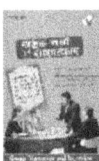

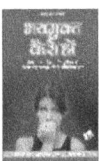

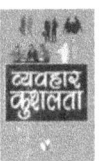

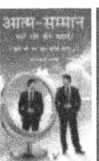

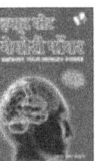

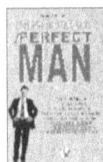

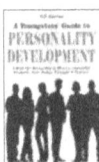

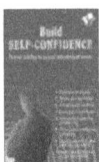

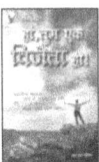

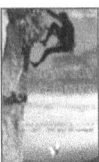

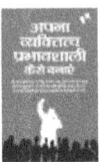

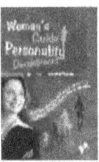

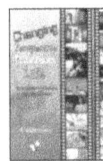

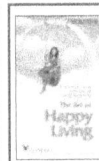

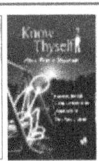

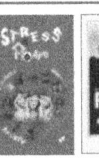

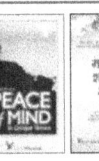

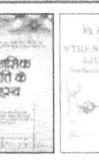

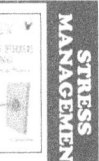

Also Available
in Kannada

Also Available
in Kannada

STRESS MANAGEMENT

All books available at www.vspublishers.com

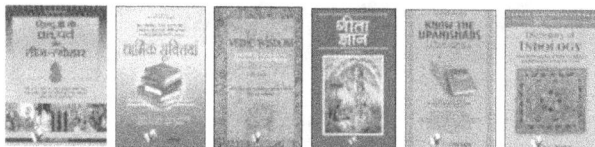

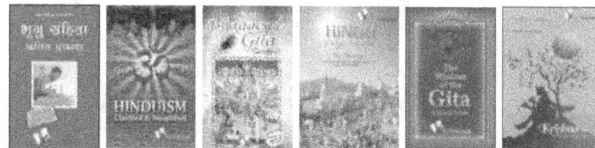

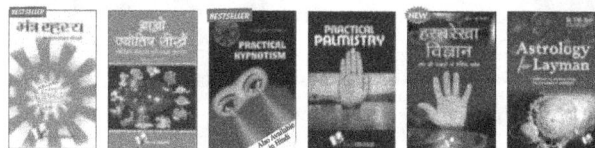

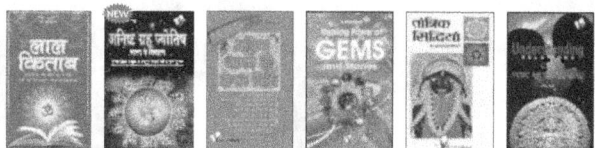

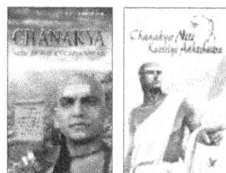

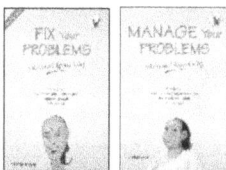

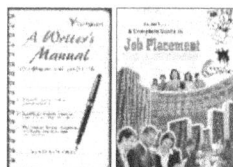

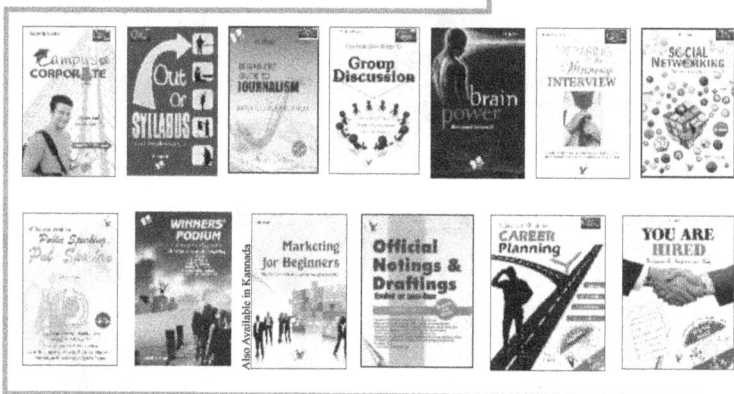

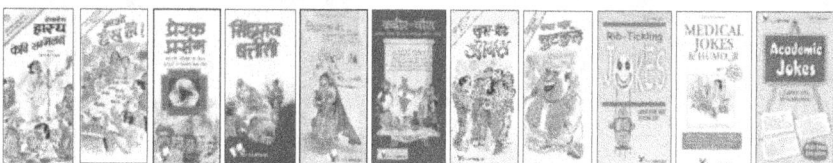

Contact us at sales@vspublishers.com

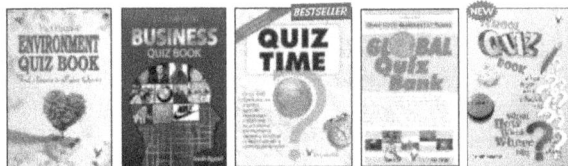
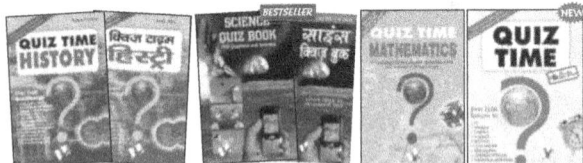
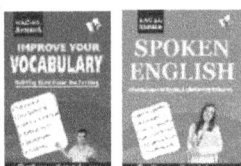
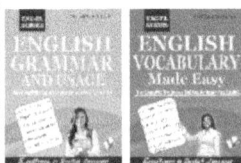
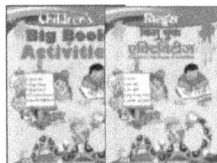
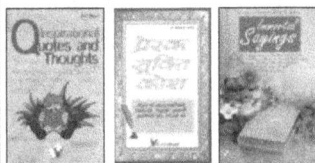
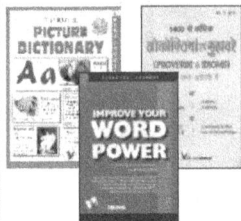
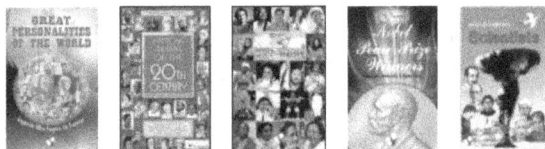
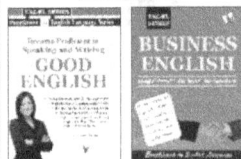
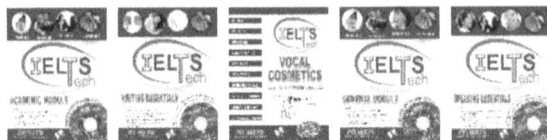
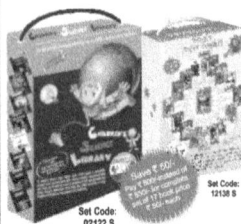
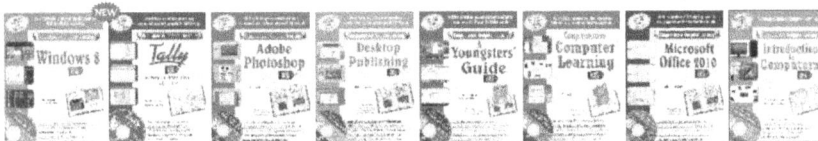

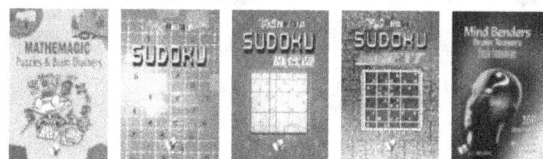

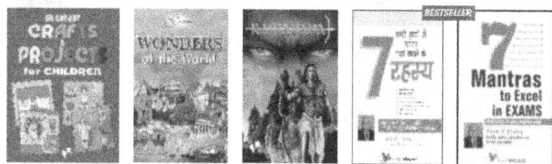

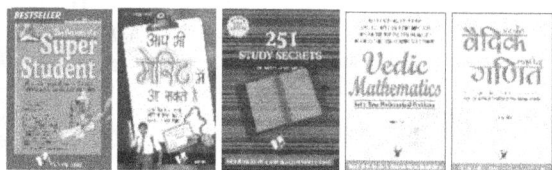

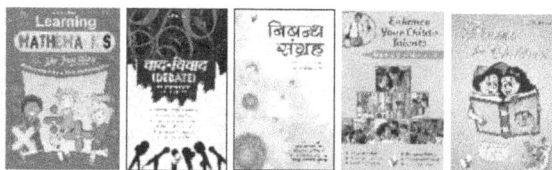

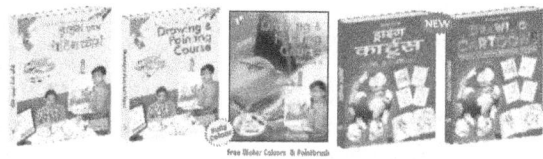

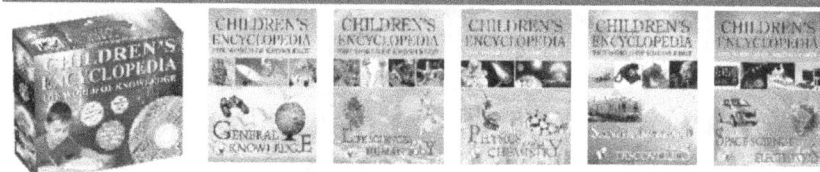

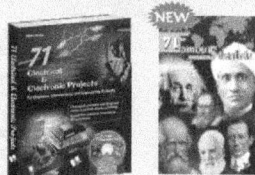

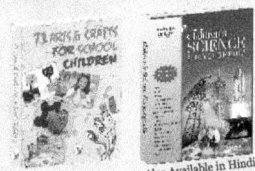

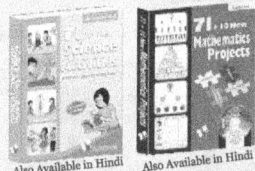

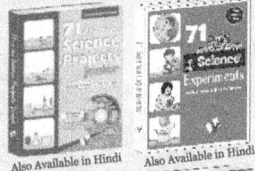

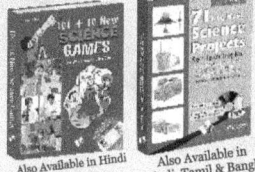

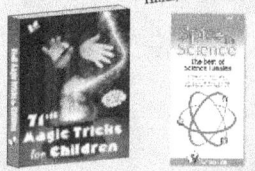

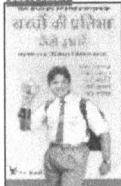 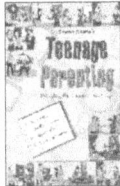 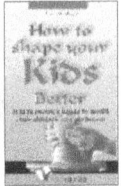 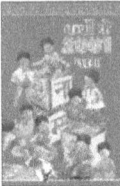 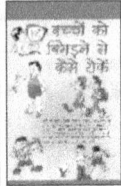 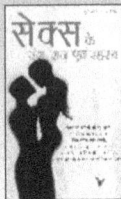 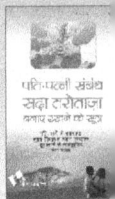
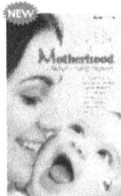 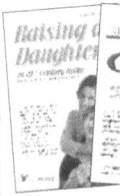 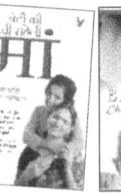 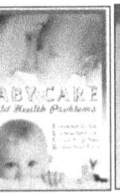 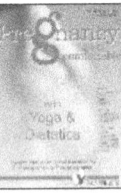 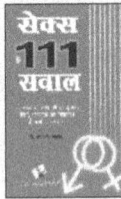 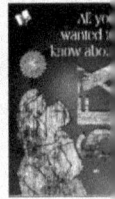
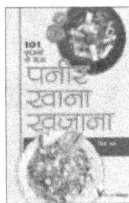 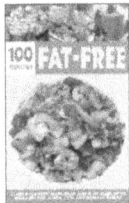 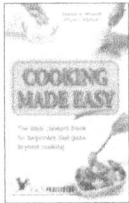 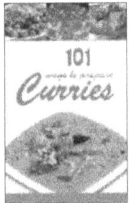 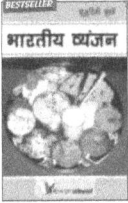 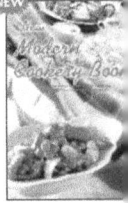
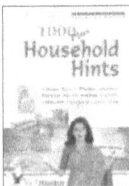 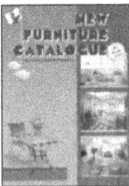 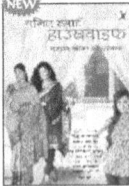 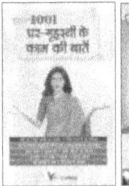 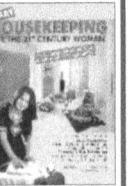 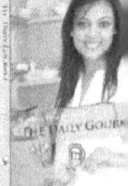
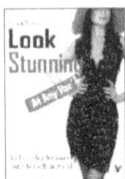 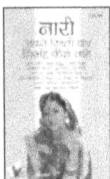 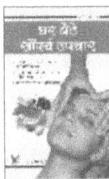 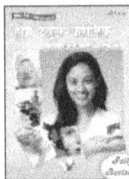 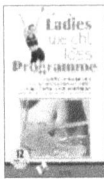 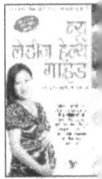
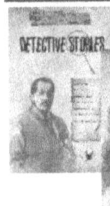 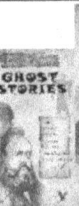 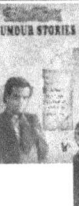 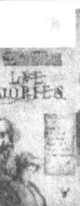 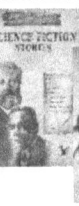 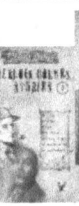 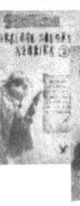 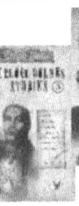  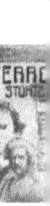

www.ingramcontent.com/pod-product-compliance
Lightning Source LLC
Chambersburg PA
CBHW071229290326
41931CB00037B/2535